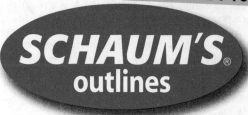

SCHAUM'S®
outlines

Medical Charting

James Keogh, RN

Instructor, New York University

Schaum's Outline Series

Mc
Graw
Hill

New York   Chicago   San Francisco   Lisbon   London   Madrid
Mexico City   Milan   New Delhi   San Juan   Seoul
Singapore   Sydney   Toronto

The **McGraw·Hill** Companies

James Keogh, RN, AAS, BSN, MBA, is a registered nurse and has written *Schaum's Outline of Pharmacology, Schaum's Outline of Nursing Laboratory and Diagnostic Tests,* and *Schaum's Outline of Medical-Surgical Nursing* and co-authored *Schaum's Outline of ECG Interpretation.* His books can be found in leading university libraries including Yale University School of Medicine, University of Pennsylvania Biomedical Library, Columbia University, Brown University, University of Medicine and Dentistry of New Jersey, Cambridge University, and Oxford University. He is a former member of the faculty of Columbia University and a member of the faculty of New York University.

Schaum's Outline of
MEDICAL CHARTING

1 2 3 4 5 6 7 8 9 10   QDB / QDB   1 0 9 8 7 6 5 4 3 2

ISBN   978-0-07-173654-1
MHID   0-07-173654-9

e-ISBN   978-0-07-173655-8
e-MHID   0-07-173655-7

McGraw-Hill books are available at special quantity discounts to use as premiums and sales promotions or for use in corporate training programs. To contact a representative please e-mail us at bulksales@mcgraw-hill.com.

This book is printed on acid-free paper.

This book is dedicated to Anne, Sandy, Joanne, Amber-Leigh Christine, Shawn, Eric, and Amy, without whose help and support this book couldn't have been written.

Contents

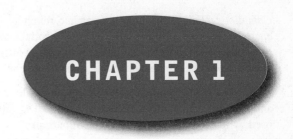

CHAPTER 1

Charting Basics

1.1 Definition

Charting is the task of creating a patient's medical record called the patient's chart. The chart is used to document a patient's healthcare and to communicate the patient's medical condition and treatment among the healthcare team.

The chart contains information describing the patient's previous and current medical conditions and the healthcare that the patient received and will receive from the healthcare team. Today the healthcare team is able to access and update patient information from computer workstations throughout the healthcare facility and from remote locations. During this transition from paper charts to electronic charts, many healthcare facilities use large loose-leaf binders to hold a patient's record.

1.1.1 The Flow of Charting

Charting begins after the patient arrives at the healthcare facility when the admitting clerk enters the patient's name, address, medical insurance, and other nonmedical information (also called "demographic information") into the chart.

The triage nurse adds the patient's medical history, current medical problem, allergies, and the patient's vital signs to the chart. This is followed by the practitioner's assessment of the patient, which is entered into the chart along with orders for medical tests, treatments, and medications.

Members of the healthcare team update the chart after carrying out each medical and nursing order required by the practitioner to further assess the patient's condition. Results of medical tests and procedures are entered into the patient's chart making the results available to the patient's healthcare team.

In addition, nurses monitor the patient 24 hours a day while the patient is in the healthcare facility. Their observations and interventions are recorded in the patient's chart several times a shift.

1.2 The Chart Is a Central Reference

The chart is also used for purposes other than providing the patient healthcare. These include:

Billing and reimbursements: Medical tests, medications, medical procedures, and other services provided to the patient that are found in the patient's medical chart are itemized on an invoice prepared by the facility's billing department based on Medicare's Diagnosis-Related Group (DRG). The invoice is submitted to the patient's insurance carrier who refers to the patient's chart to determine if care given to the patient was necessary and customary.

Compliance: Government agencies and accreditation organizations such as the Joint Commission audit patients' charts to determine if the healthcare facility and the healthcare team are in compliance with Medicare's laws and rules designed to assure that patients receive quality healthcare. If the hospital is not accredited by the Joint Commission, then the hospital will not receive reimbursement from Medicare.

Performance: Management of the healthcare facility use patients' charts to determine the cost and quality of care and whether or not care is efficiently provided to patients. Charts also serve as a performance baseline and are used by managers and staff to decide if current performance meets acceptable levels.

Education: Medical, nursing, and other interdisciplinary students (physical therapist [PT], occupational therapist [OT], nutritionist, and registered dietitian [RD]) use charts as puzzles to learn how to care for patients. Students piece together a patient's diagnosis and medical history, practitioner's orders, test results, and progress notes to understand why those orders were issued and how treatment effected the patient's condition.

Research: Medical researchers find charts contain a treasure trove of raw medical data to study and analyze. They pour over this empirical data looking for clues to improve medical science and patient care.

Legal: The patient's chart is key evidence in legal issues pertaining to a patient's medical care. Each element of the chart documents care given to the patient. Attorneys may take the position that if care isn't charted, then that care wasn't given to the patient.

1.3 Types of Charts

There are five commonly used charting systems. These are:

Narrative: The narrative charting system may be used for ambulatory care, acute care, home care, and long-term care. The narrative charting system begins with the patient health history and assessment. Progress notes (Figure 1.1) and flow sheets are entered each shift to describe the patient's status and the care that was given to the patient during the shift. The narrative chart concludes with the patient's discharge summary.

Progress Notes
08:30 Patient admitted for complaints of chest pain rated as 8 out of 10 on the pain scale. Nitroglycerin times 1 administered with relief. Resting quietly at this time.

Figure 1.1

Problem-Oriented: Problem-oriented charting may be found in acute, home, and long-term care facilities and in mental health and rehabilitation institutions. The problem-oriented charting system focuses on the patient's problems. It begins with the patient's medical history and assessment. A problem list is created based on the patient's assessment, and a care plan is developed that details how the health team is going to address each problem. Progress notes are written at each shift, and a summary is prepared for when the patient is discharged. Information is entered into the chart using SOAP, SOAPIE, SOAPIER, OLD CHARTS, or SAMPLE formats (Figures 1.2–1.6).

Progress Notes
08:30 S:"I have a lot of pain to a level 10 out of 10" O: Sitting down, grimacing, clenching fists with movement A: Abdominal pain P: Medicate for pain

Figure 1.2 SOAP.

- **S**ubjective data: what the patient says
- **O**bjective data: data based on the healthcare provider's observation and testing
- **A**ssessment data: conclusion based on subjective and objective data
- **P**lan: strategy for addressing the patient's problem

Progress Notes
08:30 P: Post operative nausea I: Medicated with Zofran 4 mg IV E: Nausea subsided:
no further complaints.

Figure 1.3 SOAPIE.

- **S**ubjective data: what the patient says
- **O**bjective data: data based on healthcare provider's observation and testing
- **A**ssessment data: conclusion based on subjective and objective data
- **P**lan: strategy for addressing the patient's problem
- **I**ntervention: the measures taken to care for the patient
- **E**valuation: the effectiveness of the intervention

Progress Notes
08:30 S:"I have a lot of pain to a level 10 out of 10" O: Sitting down, grimacing,
clenching fists with movement A: Abdominal pain P: Medicate for pain I: Medicated
with MS 2 mg IVP E: Patient pain level decreased from 10 to 3 R: Continue with plan

Figure 1.4 SOAPIER.

- **S**ubjective data: what the patient says
- **O**bjective data: data based on healthcare provider's observation and testing
- **A**ssessment data: conclusion based on subjective and objective data
- **P**lan: strategy for addressing the patient's problem
- **I**ntervention: the measures taken to care for the patient
- **E**valuation: the effectiveness of the intervention
- **R**evision: changes to the plan

Progress Notes
08:30 D: Questions regarding side effects of new medication A: Explained side effects
of new medication R: Verbalized understanding of potential side effects of new
medication

Figure 1.5 OLD CHARTS.

- **O**nset: when the problem began
- **L**ocation: location of the problem
- **D**uration: how long the problem existed
- **C**haracter: description of the problem, such as a sharp pain
- **A**lleviating and/or **A**ggravating factors: what relieves the problem and what increases the problem
- **R**adiation: progression of the problem
- **T**emporal pattern: when the problem occurs, such as every morning
- **S**ymptoms: description of the problem

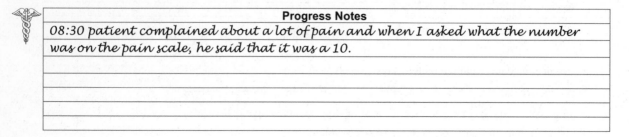

Progress Notes
08:30 patient complained about a lot of pain and when I asked what the number was on the pain scale, he said that it was a 10.

Figure 1.6 SAMPLE.

- **S**igns and symptoms: description of the problem
- **A**llergies: allergies that may or may not be involved in the problem
- **M**edications: medications the patient has taken or takes regularly
- **P**ertinent past medical history: medical history that may or may not be related to the problem
- **L**ast oral intake: anything the patient recently ingested
- **E**vents leading up to the current problem: what occurred prior to the patient noticing the problem

Problem-Intervention-Evaluation: This charting system is used mainly in acute care facilities. Problem-intervention-evaluation charting (Figure 1.7) is focused on ongoing assessment of the patient each shift. A problem list is created following the patient's history and initial assessment. The patient is then reassessed during each shift, and the results are written in progress notes and flow sheets.

Progress Notes
08:30 Complaints of pain; 10 on 1-10 pain scale

Figure 1.7

FOCUS: FOCUS charting is seen frequently in acute and long-term care facilities. FOCUS charting requires a patient's history and initial assessment. A checklist of problems (nursing diagnosis) is created, and a care plan developed. Flow sheets and progress notes are then used to document patient care. FOCUS charting (Figure 1.8) uses a data, action, and response (DAR) format.

Progress Notes
08:30 *sleepy but responsive to name and vigorous stimulation; pupils sluggish but reactive to light. Anterior lungs clear to ausculatation with rhonchi heard across lung fields; clears with coughing.*

Figure 1.8

- **D**ata: what's going on with the patient, such as the patient is having difficulty breathing

- **A**ction: measures taken, such as administration of 2 liters of oxygen using a nasal cannula

- **R**esponse: the patient's response to the action plan, such as the patient returned to normal breathing

Charting by exception: This charting method may be used in acute and long-term care facilities and is used in conjunction with the previously mentioned types of charting except for narrative charting. Narrative charting requires charting of all findings about the patient. The charting by exception documents abnormal findings compared with standards and norms established by the institution. Any deviations from these norms are entered into the chart. Charting by exception is efficient and cost-effective. The charting by exception chart contains the patient's initial assessment and problem(s). A care plan is developed to address each problem. Flow sheets and progress notes are then used to document the patient's abnormal condition.

1.4   Components of a Chart

A charting system contains these components:

Patient Information (also referred to as demographic information): Patient information consists of the patient's name, address, telephone numbers, occupation, employer, insurance carrier, and family contact information.

Patient History: Patient history provides a subjective description of the patient's health and social history. It also includes information about the medical history of the patient's family.

Episodic Information: This component documents the patient's current complaint and initial physical assessment. It answers the question what brought the patient in that day.

Psychosocial Information: Psychosocial information describes the patient's mental and development stage based on the patient's age.

Medical Orders: This component contains orders written by practitioners. These can be orders for tests, administration of medication, or procedures.

Lab Results: The lab results component identifies the laboratory tests that were performed and the results of those tests.

Test Results: There can be one or more sections of the chart for test results depending on the charting system adopted by the healthcare facility. Some charting systems will have a section for commonly performed tests such as an electrocardiogram (ECG), whereas others have one section for all tests. Test results usually contain the numeric or graphical results and a narrative that describes the examiner's findings, such as a chest x-ray report.

Progress Notes: A progress note describes an observation made by a practitioner relating to the patient's care, on a given day or time.

Nurses' Notes: Nurses' notes contain observations of the patient, interventions, and responses to interventions and are made by the patient's primary nurse.

Care Plan: The care plan describes details on how the healthcare team will address the patient's problems.

Social History: The social history records information about the patient's smoking, alcohol, and illegal drug-use history.

Legal: The legal component of the chart contains patient consent forms, living will, advanced directives, and other legal documents that direct how the patient wants to be cared for while in the healthcare facility.

Medication Administration Report (MAR): The MAR contains the record of medication ordered for the patient and when and how it was administered. Information on the MAR may be pulled from the medical orders component of the chart.

Discharge Information: The discharge information component contains a checklist of things to do when discharging the patient and a record of whether or not it was performed. It also contains instructions that the nurse must give the patient before the patient leaves the healthcare facilities.

1.5   Writing in a Chart

Writing notes in a chart tells the patient's story to members of the healthcare team and others who are involved with the patient's health.

The nursing process, referred to as ADPIE is a good approach to follow when documenting patient care. ADPIE is the acronym for assessment, diagnosis, plan, intervention, and evaluation.

Assessment: Assessment is the systematic collection of data (symptoms) reported by the patient and independently verified through observations and testing.

Diagnosis: A diagnosis is the identification of the patient's problem by looking for data clusters that lead to a pattern pointing to a problem. There are two kinds of diagnoses:

- *Medical*: A medical diagnosis is a medical determination of disease performed by a practitioner.

- *Nursing*: A nursing diagnosis is a clinical judgment of a patient and is the basis for selection of nursing interventions to achieve outcomes for which the nurse is accountable.

Plan: The plan details how the healthcare team will treat the patient. It lists who will do what and when it will be done. The plan is described in medical orders and in the patient's care plan and serves as a map to guide the healthcare team as they resolve the patient's healthcare problem.

Intervention: Intervention is carrying out the plan. Each step of the plan that is performed is documented in the chart. The time, date, route, and who administered medications are entered into the MAR (see Medication Administration Report). Test results are entered into the chart along with interpretation of those results depending on the test. All interventions must be documented in the chart. The absence of documentation means that the intervention was not performed.

Evaluation: Evaluation describes what happened after the intervention. Did the intervention resolve the patient's problems? The evaluations of interventions are documented in progress notes, nurses' notes, and flow sheets. The healthcare team may continue, modify, or terminate the plan for treating the patient depending on the evaluation.

1.6   Rules for Charting

The patient's outcomes can be affected by the accuracy of what is written in the chart. What may be simple, understandable errors such as illegible and slightly misspelled words can have a grave effect on a patient's care. Here are rules for good charting:

Everything written in a chart must be legible. This is crucial if charting entries are handwritten.

Don't assume. Illegible charting leaves others on the healthcare team one of two choices: guess at the meaning of what was written or verify it by contacting the healthcare team member who wrote it. An educated guess often overrides the time-consuming task of trying to verify the order, which can lead to fatal errors.

Does it make sense? When charting it is important that the document makes sense in terms of the patient's health. The charted information should be clearly relevant to the patient's problems, treatment plan, or intervention. The chart should only contain relative information.

Only accurate facts should be entered into the chart. Others on the healthcare team are basing their decisions on what is written in the chart. The chart should reflect what the healthcare provider personally observed and provide facts that lead to any conclusions.

Chart in a timely fashion. Ideally charting should take place at the bedside. If this is not possible, then the chart should be written immediately after leaving the patient when the information is fresh. Any delay in charting can lead to errors. Others on the healthcare team may make decisions about the patient based on outdated information.

Watch spelling! Changing one letter in a word can have an altogether different meaning and have serious repercussions for the patient. Don't guess at a spelling or phonetically spell a word. Take the time to look up the correct spelling.

Avoid abbreviations. Abbreviations save time and space when charting; however abbreviations are the source of errors because the assumption is that everyone who reads a chart knows the meanings of abbreviations.

The healthcare provider should chart only for himself. Don't chart for other members of the healthcare team. Chart only individual observations and facts.

Date and sign each entry. Begin each entry into the chart with the time and date. Document findings and then sign the entry followed by title.

Be complete in charting. Specify an intervention and evaluation for each problem that is documented. If it is charted that the patient has difficulty breathing, then the chart should also indicate what was done to solve the problem.

Use black ink. It is best to use black ink when charting. Black ink shows up better when charts are photocopied or faxed.

An incident report is *not* part of the patient's chart. An incident report must be written for errors and potential errors that occur during the patient's care (see Chapter 2).

Visitors and relatives are not authorized to see the chart. Never leave the chart open or visible to unauthorized personnel (see HIPAA in Chapter 2).

1.7 Rules for Verbal Orders

Practitioners and other members of the healthcare team who are authorized to issue orders must explicitly write those orders in the patient's chart. In some facilities, in extreme emergencies, a nurse can take verbal orders over the telephone, which is then followed up with written orders once the healthcare provider arrives at the healthcare facility.

Here are guidelines to follow when taking verbal orders:

Don't accept a verbal order if the healthcare provider is in the healthcare facility unless there is a system in place that directs the practitioner to enter the order into the computer or write the order in the chart within 24 hours of giving the verbal order.

Ask the practitioner to fax the order if possible. The fax should contain the healthcare provider's signature.

Read back the order to the practitioner to avoid errors when taking verbal orders.

Write down the order during the call. Make sure the patient is correctly identified and the right medication, dose, routine, and time are indicated if it is an order for medication.

Clarify any portion of the order that doesn't make sense. Ask the healthcare provider to spell the patient's name and names of medications. Realize that the healthcare provider can be mistaken.

Verify the order by reading it back to the healthcare provider. Also compare the verbal order to information in the patient's chart to assure that the correct patient is being addressed and that the order doesn't conflict with current orders.

Talk directly to the practitioner. Don't take verbal orders from anyone who is not authorized to issue an order.

Write the verbal order in the chart. Sign the practitioner's name followed by your name indicating that this is a verbal order. The healthcare provider must countersign the order within 24 hours.

1.8 What to Write

The objective is to clearly report on the patient's progress using as few words as possible. The writing provides other members of the healthcare team facts about the patient that help them continue caring for the patient.

It is critical to chart facts and not opinions. For example, "had a good day" or "did not appear to be in that much pain" are opinions, not facts. On the other hand, "patient reported a pain of 2 on a scale of 0 to 10" is fact.

Charting "physician was called" is a fact; however "when I called the physician about this patient, he sounded tired and not interested in what I had to say" is an opinion.

Avoid writing words that could defame someone. Charting is not the place to attack the good name and reputation of the patient or anyone on the healthcare team.

Keep charting to a minimum amount of words while conveying important facts about the patient.

A common trick used by experienced nurses is to draw a mental picture of the patient's problem and then describe that image in the chart. Let's say that the task is to describe a wound. Picture the wound and then describe the wound in the chart, such as "large abdominal dressing intact with 1 cm of red/brown wound drainage noted."

Another trick is to think logically and systematically when charting. Use a top-down approach and describe each system completely before moving on to the next system.

1.9 Fixing Errors

Expect to make errors when writing in a chart because it happens to everyone. Typically, information is added on a page that already contains information entered by others on the healthcare team; therefore simply ripping up the page and starting over isn't an option when an error is entered on the chart.

Instead draw a *single* line through the error and initial above the line. Don't cover up the error with Wite-Out or heavily cross out the text making it unreadable. The error must be legible and clearly indicated as an error. Making the error illegible might lead someone to believe that the error is being concealed.

Solved Problems

1.1   When does charting begin?

Charting begins after the patient arrives at the healthcare facility when the admitting clerk enters the patient's name, address, medical insurance, and other nonmedical information into the chart

1.2   What are the purposes for charting?

- Billing and reimbursement
- Compliance
- Performance management
- Education
- Research
- Legal record

1.3   What is a narrative chart?

The narrative charting system is used for ambulatory care, acute care, home care, and long-term care. The narrative charting system begins with the patient health history and assessment. Progress notes and flow sheets are entered each shift to describe the patient's status and the care that was given to the patient during the shift. The narrative chart concludes with the patient's discharge summary.

1.4   What is a problem-oriented chart?

The problem-oriented charting system focuses on the patient's problems. It begins with the patient's medical history and assessment. A problem list is created based on the patient's assessment and a care plan is developed that details how the health team is going to address each problem. Progress notes are written at each shift and a discharge summary is prepared for when the patient is discharged

1.5   What is SOAP?

- **S**ubjective data: what the patient says
- **O**bjective data: data based on observation and testing
- **A**ssessment data: conclusion based on subjective and objective data
- **P**lan: strategy for addressing the patient's problem

1.6   What is SOAPIE?

- **S**ubjective data: what the patient says
- **O**bjective data: data based on observation and testing
- **A**ssessment data: conclusion based on subjective and objective data
- **P**lan: strategy for addressing the patient's problem
- **I**ntervention: the measures taken to care for the patient
- **E**valuation: the effectiveness of the intervention

1.7   What is SOAPIER?

- **S**ubjective data: what the patient says
- **O**bjective data: data based on observation and testing
- **A**ssessment data: conclusion based on subjective and objective data
- **P**lan: strategy for addressing the patient's problem

- Intervention: the measures taken to care for the patient

- Evaluation: the effectiveness of the intervention

- Revision: changes to the plan

1.8   What is OLD CHART?

- **O**nset: when the problem occurred

- **L**ocation: location of the problem

- **D**uration: how long the problem existed

- **C**haracter: description of the problem, such as a sharp pain

- **A**lleviating and **A**ggravating factors: what relieves the problem and what increases the problem

- **R**adiation: progression of the problem

- **T**emporal pattern: when does the problem occur, such as every morning

- **S**ymptoms: description of the problem

1.9   What is SAMPLE?

- **S**igns and symptoms: description of the problem

- **A**llergies: allergies that may or may not be involved in the problem

- **M**edications: medications the patient has taken or regularly takes

- **P**ertinent past medical history: medical history that may or may not be related to the problem

- **L**ast oral intake: anything that the patient recently ingested

- **E**vents leading up to the current problem: what occurred prior to the patient noticing the problem

1.10   What is problem-intervention-evaluation charting?

This charting system is used mainly in acute care facilities. Problem-intervention-evaluation charting is focused on ongoing assessment of the patient each shift. A problem list is created following the patient's history and initial assessment. The patient is then reassessed during each shift, and the results are written in progress notes and flow sheets.

1.11   What is FOCUS charting?

FOCUS charting is seen frequently in acute and long-term care facilities. FOCUS charting requires a patient's history and initial assessment. A checklist of problems (nursing diagnosis) is created, and a care plan developed. Flow sheets and progress notes are then used to document patient care.

1.12   What is the DAR format?

FOCUS charting uses a data, action, and response (DAR) format.

- **D**ata: what's going on with the patient, such as breathing difficulty

- **A**ction: measures taken such as administration of 2 liters of oxygen using a nasal cannula

- **R**esponse: patient's response to action plan, such as return to normal breathing

1.13 What is charting by exception?

The charting by exception documents abnormal findings compared with standards and norms established by the institution. Any deviations from these are entered into the chart.

1.14 What is episodic information?

This component documents the patient's current complaint and initial physical assessment. It answers the question what brought the patient in that day.

1.15 What is social history information?

Social history information records information about the patient's use of smoking materials, alcohol, and illegal drugs currently and in the past.

1.16 What are medical orders?

The medical orders component contains orders written by healthcare providers. These can be orders for tests, administration of medication, or procedures.

1.17 What are progress notes?

A progress note describes an observation made by a healthcare provider, such as a practitioner, relating to the patient's care on a given day or time.

1.18 What are nurses' notes?

Nurse's notes contain observations of the patient made by the patient's primary nurse.

1.19 What is a care plan?

The care plan describes details on how the healthcare team will address the patient's problems.

1.20 What is the MAR?

Medication Administration Report (MAR): The MAR contains the record of medication ordered for the patient and when it was administered.

1.21 What is discharge information?

The discharge information component contains a checklist of things to do when discharging the patient and a record of whether or not it was performed. It also contains instructions that the nurse must give the patient before the patient leaves the healthcare facilities.

1.22 What is meant by chart only for yourself?

Don't chart for other members of the healthcare team. Chart only personal observations and facts.

1.23 What is an incident report?

An incident report is *not* part of the patient's chart. An incident report must be written for errors and potential errors that occur during the patient's care.

1.24   What is a verbal order?

Practitioners and other members of the healthcare team who are authorized to issue orders must explicitly write those orders in the patient's chart. In extreme emergencies, a nurse can take verbal orders over the telephone, which is then followed up with written orders once the healthcare provider arrives at the healthcare facility.

1.25   What is the proper way to correct an error in a chart?

Draw a single line through the error and initial above the line with the correction.

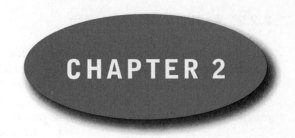

CHAPTER 2

Charting Legalities

2.1   Definition

The content of the patient's chart is the legal record of what did and did not occur in the treatment of the patient. The contents of the patients' charts weighs heavily in the decisions of judges and jurors who determine facts in malpractice actions. Words written in the patient's chart can make the difference between a successful malpractice lawsuit and dismissal of the case.

A chart that conforms to best healthcare practices and standards implies that the patient received a high level of care from the healthcare team. Conversely, a chart with poor or incomplete documentation infers that the patient received a substandard level of care.

2.2   A Patient's Legal Medical Record

The patient's chart is a confidential record protected by ethical and legal regulations that define how it can be used and by whom. The goal of these regulations is to give patients control of their healthcare information and to limit access to patient information to those who provide care to the patient. This includes physicians, nurses, medical insurers, and administrators who are involved in billing, reimbursement, and managing the healthcare facility, as well as other interdisciplinary personnel caring for the patient (PT, OT, Registered Dietician).

2.2.1   Limited Access to Medical Records

Each person who is involved with the patient's care is permitted to access just the patient's data that is necessary to deliver his or her service—not access to the complete chart. For example, a pharmacist needs information about the patient to provide proper medication but doesn't need to know the patient's address or billing information.

Patient confidentiality extends to discussions about the patient with others who are not directly involved in the patient's care, including casual conversations with colleagues. Information about a patient may be shared with colleagues but the patient's identity must remain confidential. Nurses can ask a colleague for suggestions on how to intervene in specific conditions that affects a patient without revealing the identity of the patient.

2.2.2 An Unknowing Violation

Patient confidentiality is violated if the colleague can piece together information given by the nurse. Suppose the nurse asks a colleague about interventions for a patient with prostrate problems. If there is only one male patient in the unit who is 50 years old or older, then it is easy to determine the patient to whom the nurse refers.

Other clues to the patient's identity are age, gender, diagnosis, practitioner (if the practitioner has only one patient on the unit), unusual event (i.e., one patient on the unit acted out), nationality, race, and handicap.

2.2.3 Protecting Patient's Rights

Guard against unauthorized access to the patient's chart while the patient is in the unit. Immediately challenge anyone who requests a chart or who is seen reviewing the chart if that person is not involved with the patient's care.

Protect the patient's identity from public display. This becomes a balancing act between the need to protect patient confidentiality and the need for members of the healthcare team to identify the patient.

For example, some healthcare facilities post staff's patient assignments on a large board near the nurses' station or at the entrance to the unit. This enables the staff to quickly identify who is responsible for a patient's care. Only the nurse's first name, the patient's initials, and the room number may be listed. More details might be available on a clipboard at the nurse's station.

Using room and bed numbers to identify a patient is a violation of the Joint Commission. Some facilities use the patient's first name and first initial of the last name.

A similar problem exists with identifying charts if the facility doesn't use computerized charting; even with computerized charting, there is always a paper chart. Paper charts are usually stored in large loose-leaf binders at the nurses' station or in a mobile cart used during rounds. The patient's identity appears on the spine of the loose-leaf binder. Facilities commonly label the chart with the room and bed number.

2.2.4 Health Insurance Portability and Accountability Act (HIPAA)

The Health Insurance Portability and Accountability Act (HIPAA) is the primary legislation governing the use of medical records. HIPAA establishes rules for securing and managing a patient's healthcare records as well as coding and reimbursements.

Practitioners are required to inform their patients about HIPAA's privacy requirements and ask patients to sign an acknowledgement that they were notified by the practitioner. Patients also must be asked to sign a consent allowing the practitioner to share the patient's medical records for routine medical care.

In keeping with the goal of patient confidentiality, HIPAA requires that patient information be disclosed on a need-to-know basis. The practitioner must explain to patients how they maintain the required patient confidentiality.

2.3 Limit Legal Liability

The patient's chart describes the patient's condition, diagnosis, and care while the patient was in the healthcare facility and is therefore the cornerstone to malpractice actions. Inaccurate or incomplete documentation indicates to a judge and jury that the patient received below standard care.

The best defense against a malpractice suit is accurately documenting patient care. Chart exactly the patient's assessment and treatment in terms that leave no doubt as to what occurred. Describe the patient's problem (assessment), what was done to address the problem (intervention), and how the patient reacted (outcome). Excluding any of these leaves the chart incomplete and open to speculation by attorneys, judges, and jurors. If it isn't charted, then it didn't happen.

2.3.1   Targets of Malpractice

The purpose of charting is to provide factual information about the patient to members of the healthcare team. Providing consistent and comprehensive information is also the best way to defend a malpractice case. Chart anything that might be important in malpractice litigation.

Standards for charting are defined by:

- *Nurse Practice Acts*: Defines the scope of practice for nurses
- *American Nurses Association (ANA)*: Provides standards used to accredit the healthcare facility
- *The facility's own policy*: Defines individual facility's own standards and typically incorporates ANA standards

Malpractice attorneys focus on common errors that occur in charting and then exploit them as proof that malpractice has occurred.

Tips to avoid these errors:

Correct errors in the chart immediately, otherwise the error can lead to additional errors.

Don't make errors in the chart illegible. The assumption will be that there was an attempt to hide something. Draw a single line through the error and initial it using the same black pen that was used to write the incorrect information in the chart. This shows that the error was recognized and corrected immediately.

Don't chart in advance. Although doing so saves time, there is a risk of possible distraction and not providing the treatment.

Don't enter the incorrect time. Patient load sometimes prevents providing treatment when it is scheduled. This can have serious ramifications, especially when administering medication.

Don't write critical comments or opinions in the chart. Simply write the objective facts using acceptable medical terminology and let the reader draw a conclusion based on those facts.

Don't leave any blank space between chart entry and signature. This leaves the opportunity for someone else to add information to what has been charted. Draw a line through the space if leaving a space cannot be avoided.

Enter verbal orders in the chart immediately and make sure that the practitioner signs them. Verbal orders that don't appear in the chart are considered not ordered.

Don't skip lines when charting. All information must be on consecutive lines.

Always use black ink. Attempts to alter the chart will easily be noticed.

Don't allude in the chart to the filing of an incident report.

Make sure to perform a complete assessment of the patient and chart results. Failure to do so can be construed as breach of duty.

Avoid mentioning other patients in the chart because this violates patient confidentiality.

Always document the patient's response and comments by placing the patient's exact words in quotations.

Make sure to enter accurate information into the correct patient's chart. It is best to take a 10-second time-out to collect thoughts before writing anything in the chart.

Don't carry out orders that seem questionable. Document any calls to the practitioner for clarification for the specific order. Be sure to note the date and time.

Always chart instructions given to the patient when the patient is discharged and chart whether or not the patient understood those discharge instructions. Chart if the patient was not able to demonstrate or verbalize the discharge instructions and chart intervention to re-educate the patient.

Avoid using words that imply that an error occurred.

2.3.2 Elements of Malpractice

The chart is a key element that determines if a malpractice action is successful. The court and jurors examine the chart to determine if the patient received the standard care from the healthcare team. The standard tested in the courts is whether or not a reasonable and equally trained member of the healthcare team having similar experience would have acted the same as the defendant in caring for the patient.

The patient's attorney sets out to prove that the patient was injured (damage) because of the medical team's action (causation) or inaction (breach of duty) which demonstrates negligence when caring for the patient. That is, the healthcare team did something that should not have been performed or didn't do something that should have been performed according to standard care.

Malpractice is a form of negligence that stipulates that a professional did not act reasonably and in good faith while performing a service to another person. That is, did not respond the way another professional may have responded.

Whether or not a procedure was malpractice depends on the following factors:

- Did the patient consent to the procedure?

- Was the patient informed of the risks of performing the procedure?

- Did the practitioner order the procedure?

- Was the nurse who performed the procedure trained, validated, licensed, and authorized by the healthcare facility to perform the procedure?

- Did the nurse adhere to the standards when performing the procedure?

If the answers are yes, then malpractice didn't occur. Answering no to any of these questions raises the question of malpractice because there is a failure to meet the standard of care that the patient is entitled to receive.

Attorneys compare the patient's chart, the facility's policies, the healthcare team's background and standards established by legal and accrediting organizations to the treatment that the patient received to prove their case of malpractice.

2.4 An Incident Report

An incident report documents a serious exception to normal procedures that may be dangerous or may lead to potential litigation. The policies of the healthcare facility describe situations when an incident report must be filed with the risk management department or the appropriate department within the facility. Never place an incident report in the patient's chart, otherwise the incident report can be used as evidence in litigation.

The risk management department conducts its own investigation and reports the results to the healthcare facility's attorney and insurance carrier. The situation leading up to and the handling of the incident are reviewed by management in order to improve procedures depending on the nature of the incident.

Each person who is involved in the incident, including those who witnessed all or part of the incident, should file an incident report that describes the facts of the incident according to their first-hand observations.

In writing the incident report, the healthcare provider should:

- Write the incident report on forms provided by the healthcare facility. Use additional pages if needed.

- Make sure to identify the patient, the time, and place of the incident, and what was done once the incident came to light.

- Describe how the incident affected the patient.

- Don't leave blank spaces on the incident report. Draw a single line through any blank spaces. This prevents anyone else from inserting facts to the writer's incident report.

- Never write observations on someone else's incident report.

- Write only facts that are personally identified. If the healthcare provider didn't see it, then she shouldn't write about it—no assumptions or opinions. Let others draw a conclusion from the facts.

- Make sure facts in the chart coincide with facts in the incident report.

- Specify what was done upon encountering the incident.

- Write in quotations whatever the patient or others say to the healthcare provider.

- Avoid blaming anyone for the incident. Let the facts speak for themselves.

2.5 Other Legal Documents

The chart contains legal documents of which the most common are informed consent, advance directives, and a refusal of treatment.

- *Informed Consent*: The informed consent authorizes the medical team to perform a specific procedure or administer a specific treatment to the patient.

- *Advance Directive*: An advance directive tells the healthcare team the patient's wishes for care should the patient become incapacitated and unable to communicate.

- *Refusal of Treatment*: Refusal of treatment acknowledges that the patient is rejecting prescribed medical care.

Each legal document must be:

- Explained to the patient

- Discussed in terms of risks and benefits

- Presented, to include alternative options, including the option of doing nothing

- Signed by the patient in order for the legal document to take effect

The patient must be legally competent to sign the document and have the capability to fully comprehend the contents of the document. Hospital policies and laws determine legal competency. Assess comprehension of the document by asking the patient to repeat in the patient's own words the content of the document. If the patient can't explain the proposed treatment, then stop. Further explanation is needed from the practitioner.

Once the practitioner is confident that the patient understands, then the patient is asked to sign the document, and the practitioner countersigns it as a witness to the patient's signature.

Only patients who are legally competent can sign the document, otherwise a guardian such as a parent or court-appointed representative can sign on behalf of the patient.

2.5.1 Informed Consent

An informed consent authorizes the healthcare team to perform procedures on the patient. The patient must consent before any procedure is performed, including routine procedures that are covered by the general consent form signed when the patient is admitted to the healthcare facility.

Consent for routine procedures such as inserting a urinary catheter can be given orally. However, the patient must still be told why the practitioners wants the procedure performed, the benefits and risks associated with it, and options to performing the procedure.

There are two situations when a signed informed consent is not necessary. These are in an emergency and if the patient isn't interested in hearing about the treatment.

When asking for an informed consent, consider the following:

- The practitioner is responsible to have the patient sign the informed consent. It is not the nurse's responsibility.

- The practitioner must provide the patient with information necessary for the patient to make an informed decision to either undergo the prescribed treatment or to opt for alternative treatment or no treatment at all.

- The nurse advocates for the patient to make sure that a consent form has been signed by the patient.

- The nurse asks the patient if the patient understood the practitioner's explanation about the diagnoses, prescribed treatment, and the risks involved in the treatment.

- The nurse asks if the practitioner discussed alternative treatments and the risk for each.

- The nurse encourages the patient to ask questions, and then the nurse answers them or has the practitioner return to further explain the proposed procedure.

- The nurse is responsible for making sure that the patient understands the procedure.

- The nurse might be asked to witness the patient signing the consent form. If this happens, the nurse also signs the consent form as a witness.

- It is critical that the patient also understands that the consent is only for a particular treatment.

- Current treatment continues even if the patient doesn't sign the consent form.

- The patient will still be offered future treatment regardless of if the consent form is signed.

- The patient must be told that consent can be withdrawn at anytime even after the consent form is signed.

- The patient can simply tell the practitioner to stop, and treatment will be stopped.

- Patients must sign the consent form of their own free will based on all the options presented to them by the practitioner.

- Failure to objectively present the benefits and risks of all the treatment alternatives can be construed as coercion and might nullify the signed consent form.

- The healthcare team might be committing a battery if treatment is given without a valid, signed consent form.

- Once the consent form is signed and countersigned as witness to the signature, the consent form is placed in the patient's chart.

- The nurse documents in the nurse's notes that the patient signed or refused to sign the consent form after the treatment was explained by the practitioner.

- The nurse documents that the patient refused to sign the consent form and explicitly describes his actions and the patient's response. The nurse documents the patient's actual words using quotations and documents what he did after the patient refused to sign, such as contacting the nurse manager and the practitioner, and the steps taken to prevent the treatment from beginning.

2.5.2 Advance Directives

An advance directive is a legal document signed by the patient that gives the healthcare team instructions about the kind of life-sustaining care the patient desires, should the patient be unable to convey his or her wishes.

Any legally competent adult can create an advance directive.

An advance directive must be signed and the signature witnessed.

Terms of the advance directive must comply with legal restrictions, which may define basic care (i.e., nutrients) that must be given to all patients regardless of their wishes.

The patient can request not to be resuscitated if he or she experiences cardiac arrest or respiratory arrest, or to be disconnected from life-supporting equipment if there is no hope for the patient's survival.

The patient can change the advance directive at any time by telling the practitioner that he or she no longer wants the advance directive enforced. The healthcare facility will have a policy describing how to document the patient's request to change the advance directive.

An advance directive signed prior to being admitted to the healthcare facility must be copied, and the copy must be placed in the patient's chart and documented in the nurse's notes.

If the patient doesn't have an advance directive, then the healthcare facility usually can provide an advance directive form that the patient can use to indicate his or her wishes.

The nurse might be required to witness the patient's signature. If so, then the nurse should document the patient's mental state in the nurse's notes. This becomes evidence that the patient was competent at the time the advance directive was created.

Failure to comply with terms of an advance directive can expose the healthcare team to legal action by the patient or the patient's family.

The advance directive is followed only when the patient is comatose—unable to speak for him or herself.

There are two types of advance directives:

Living Will: A living will specifies the kind of care the patient wants to receive if he or she becomes incapacitated requiring extraordinary measures (i.e., feeding tube, ventilator) to sustain the patient's life.

Durable Power of Attorney: A durable power of attorney designates a person to make healthcare decisions for the patient if the patient becomes unable to make decisions for himself or herself. Contact information in the durable power of attorney may be outdated unless it was recently created; the nurse should make sure she can contact the designated person.

Do Not Resuscitate (DNR) is an order written by a practitioner if the patient specifies in an advance directive that the patient does not want to be resuscitated should the patient arrest.

   Many hospitals have variations of the DNR order:

Do Not Intubate (DNI) is a DNR order that enables the practitioner to take lifesaving measures up until the point of intubation.

Slow Code: A slow code is less than a full effort to recover the patient if the patient arrests. This is based on the patient's poor condition. The practitioner who orders a slow code and the healthcare team who performs a slow code are committing an illegal act. Barring a DNR order, the healthcare team must make an all-out effort to resuscitate the patient.

Here are some factors to consider for a DNR:

It is important for the practitioner to review the patient's advance directive if the patient is at risk for becoming comatose or arresting.

The practitioner will write a DNR order if the practitioner feels that the patient understands the impact of the DNR order.

The practitioner may choose not to write the DNR order. If this happens, the nurse needs to document this in the nurse's notes.

Don't call a code if the patient has a DNR order.

Some healthcare facilities clearly mark DNR on the spine of the patient's chart that has a DNR provision in his or her advance directive so that the healthcare team can respond appropriately in an emergency.

The DNR order should be reviewed with the patient frequently and particularly when the patient's condition changes, especially for the better. The patient may want to rescind the DNR request. Healthcare facilities have policies that specify how to handle a DNR order.

A DNR order must be reviewed and renewed by the practitioner every 72 hours.

A verbal DNR order is not acceptable. Every DNR order must be written.

Always let the nurse manager, practitioner, the healthcare facility's legal department, or other appropriate department handle advance directives issues.

2.5.3   Refusal of Treatment

A legally competent patient has the right to refuse treatment and can request to be discharged against medical advice (AMA). Healthcare facilities typically have a Refuse Treatment form and a Discharge Against Medical Advice form which the patient is requested to sign releasing the healthcare team from liability.

    The patient can refuse complete treatment or an aspect of the treatment such as insertion of a urinary catheter. When this occurs, the practitioner is required to explain to the patient the benefits of the treatment and the risk of not undergoing treatment. Once the practitioner is convinced the patient is making an informed decision, then the patient is presented with the Refuse Treatment form.

Refuse Treatment Form: The Refuse Treatment form describes the patient's diagnosis and treatment and acknowledges that the practitioner explained the risk of failing to undergo treatment. The patient is asked to sign the form, which is countersigned by a witness. The form is then placed in the patient's chart.

Discharge Against Medical Advice Form: The Discharge Against Medical Advice form must contain the patient's own words stating that he wants to leave and understands the risk of leaving. Furthermore, the form must also identify the practitioner who explained the risk to the patient. Although the patient is free to leave the healthcare facility, the healthcare team is required to give the patient written directions for follow-up medical care, such as at the clinic, and notify the patient's family that the patient is leaving against medical advice and may require additional support at home. It is important to document what the recommended follow-up support is, which relatives were notified, where the patient is going after being discharged, and who accompanied the patient leaving the healthcare facility.

There should be documentation in the nurse's notes whenever a patient refuses treatment or is discharged against medical advice. The notes should record the patient's mental state and exact words and what happened after the patient made the request.

    The healthcare provider can't force the patient to sign any form. Healthcare facilities have policies on how to respond to such situations. Typically, the practitioner and another member of the healthcare team will witness the patient's refusal and then note that in the patient's chart (nurse's notes or progress notes). Some healthcare facilities ask a member of the patient's family to sign the form as confirmation of the patient's intent.

    The practitioner should explain to the patient each aspect of the planned treatment immediately after the patient is admitted. Should the patient refuse the planned treatment, the practitioner might provide alternatives to the treatment plan.

2.6   Patient Elopement

Patient elopement occurs when the patient simply leaves the healthcare facility without telling anyone. When this occurs, the healthcare provider should take the following steps to locate the patient:

- Contact security
- Contact his or her supervisor

- Call the patient's family

- Notify the police

- This entire event should be documented objectively and chronologically. It should include when and how it was discovered that the patient was missing and the response to the situaion and who and when the call for assistance was made and what the response was. The event should be recorded so that anyone reading it is able to retrace every step.

2.7 Charting and Patient Rights

Here are a few things to keep in mind when working with a chart and patient information:

- Patients have the right to see their charts and other parts of their medical records.

- Patients can receive a copy of their medical records.

- Patients can ask for amendments to their medical records.

- Patients have the right to restrict the kind of information that is shared and with whom it is shared.

- It is important to develop a nurse-patient relationship to address any perceived dissatisfaction with care before the patient seeks legal remedies.

Solved Problems

2.1   What is a patient's chart?

The patient's chart is the legal record of what did and did not occur in the treatment of the patient.

2.2   What impact does a chart have in a malpractice action?

A chart that conforms to best healthcare practices and standards implies that the patient received a high level of care from the healthcare team. Conversely, a chart with poor or incomplete documentation infers that the patient received a substandard level of care.

2.3   What determines who has access to a patient's medical record?

Each person who is involved with the patient's care is permitted to access just the patient's data that is necessary to deliver his or her service—not access to the complete chart.

2.4   Who is affected by patient confidentiality?

Patient confidentiality extends to discussions about the patient with others who are not directly involved in the patient's care, including casual conversations with colleagues. Information about a patient can be shared with colleagues as long as the patient's identity remains confidential.

2.5   What is a common way patient confidentiality is violated?

Patient confidentiality is violated if a colleague can piece together information given by the nurse.

2.6 What should a healthcare provider do if asked for information about the patient?

He or she should immediately challenge anyone who requests a chart or who is seen reviewing the chart if that person is not involved with the patient's care.

2.7 Is it permissible to use the patient room and bed number to identify a patient?

Using room and bed numbers to identify a patient is a violation of the Joint Commission.

2.8 What law establishes rules for securing and managing a patient's healthcare records?

Health Insurance Portability and Accountability Act (HIPAA).

2.9 How can a patient's medical records be shared by a practitioner for routine medical care?

Patients must be asked to sign a consent allowing the practitioner to share the patient's medical records for routine medical care.

2.10 What guideline should be used for releasing a patient's medical records?

In keeping with the goal of patient confidentiality, HIPAA requires that patient information be disclosed on a need-to-know basis.

2.11 What is the best defense against malpractice action?

The best defense against a malpractice suit is accurately documenting patient care.

2.12 What would prevent attorneys, judges, and jurors from speculating about patient care in a malpractice action?

The healthcare provider should chart exactly the patient's assessment and treatment in terms that leave no doubt as to what occurred. He or she should describe the patient's problem (assessment), what was done to address the problem (intervention), and how the patient reacted (outcome). Excluding any of these components leaves the chart incomplete and open to speculation by attorneys, judges, and jurors. If it isn't charted, then it didn't happen.

2.13 Who or what defines charting standards?

- Nurse Practice Acts: Defines the scope of practice for nurses.

- American Nurses Association (ANA): Provides standards used to accredit the healthcare facility.

- The facility's own policy: Defines individual facility's own standards and typically incorporate ANA standards.

2.14 How can common errors that occur in charting be avoided?

- Correct errors in the chart immediately.

- Don't make errors in the chart illegible.

- Don't chart in advance.

- Don't enter the incorrect time.

- Don't write critical comments or opinions in the chart.

- Don't leave any blank space between an entry and that writer's signature.

- Enter verbal orders in the chart immediately and make sure that the practitioner signs them.
- Don't skip lines when charting.
- Always use black ink.
- Don't allude in the chart to the filing of an incident report.
- Perform a complete assessment of the patient and chart results.
- Avoid mentioning other patients in the chart because this violates patient confidentiality.
- Always document the patient's response and comments by placing the patient's exact words in quotations.
- Enter accurate information into the correct patient's chart.
- Don't carry out orders that are questionable.
- Always chart instructions given to the patient when the patient is discharged and chart whether or not the patient understood those discharge instructions.
- Avoid using words that imply that an error occurred.

2.15 What is the patient's attorney's goal in a malpractice action?

The patient's attorney sets out to prove that the patient was injured (damage) because of the medical team's action (causation) or inaction (breach of duty) which demonstrates negligence when caring for the patient. That is, the healthcare team did something that should not have been performed or didn't do something that should have been performed according to standard care.

2.16 What is malpractice?

Malpractice is a form of negligence that stipulates that a professional did not act reasonably and in good faith while performing a service to another person—that is, did not respond the way another professional may have responded.

2.17 What factors influence malpractice?

- Did the patient consent to the procedure?
- Was the patient informed of the risks of performing the procedure?
- Did the practitioner order the procedure?
- Was the nurse who performed the procedure trained, validated, licensed, and authorized by the healthcare facility to perform the procedure?
- Did the nurse have reason to believe that the equipment was sterile and working properly?
- Did the nurse adhere to the standards when performing the procedure?

2.18 What does the patient's attorney compare the patient's chart to?

Attorneys compare the patient's chart, the facility's policies, the healthcare team's background, and standards established by legal and accrediting organizations to the treatment that the patient received to prove their case of malpractice.

2.19 What is an incident report?

An incident report documents a serious exception to normal procedures that may be dangerous or may lead to potential litigation.

2.20　What should a healthcare provider do when writing an incident report?

- Write an incident report on forms provided by the healthcare facility. Use additional pages if needed.

- Make sure to identify the patient, the time and place of the incident, and what was done once the healthcare provider became aware of the incident.

- Describe how the incident affected the patient.

- Don't leave blank spaces on the incident report. Draw a single line through any blank spaces. This prevents anyone from inserting facts to the incident report after the healthcare provider completes his or her entry.

- Don't write observations on someone else's incident report.

- Write only facts that were identified. The healthcare provider should write only what was observed—no assumptions or opinions. Let others draw a conclusion from the facts.

- Make sure facts in the chart coincide with facts in the incident report.

- Specify what was done when the incident was encountered.

- Write in quotations whatever the patient or others say.

- Don't blame anyone for the incident. Let the facts speak for themselves.

2.21　What is an informed consent?

The informed consent authorizes the medical team to perform a specific procedure or administer a specific treatment to the patient.

2.22　What is an advance directive?

An advance directive tells the healthcare team the patient's wishes for care should the patient become incapacitated and unable to communicate.

2.23　What is refusal of treatment?

Refusal of treatment acknowledges that the patient is rejecting prescribed medical care.

2.24　What must be done with a legal document before the patient signs the document?

- The document must be explained to the patient.

- The benefits and risks must be discussed.

- Alternative options must be presented, including the option of doing nothing.

- The document must be signed by the patient in order for the legal document to take effect.

2.25　What happens when the patient is not legally competent to sign a document?

Only patients who are legally competent can sign the document, otherwise a guardian such as a parent or court-appointed representative can sign on behalf of the patient.

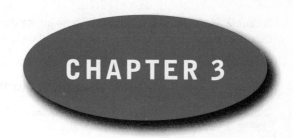

CHAPTER 3

Charting Medication and Routine

3.1 Definition

Charting medication and routine medical care is a critical aspect of charting because the healthcare provider's words become part of the patient's official record that will be used by other members of the healthcare team to decide the best course of treatment for the patient.

Charting must be thorough and complete, yet brief. That is, the chart is a news report about the patient rather than the patient's life story.

Furthermore, the patient's health insurer may base reimbursements to the healthcare facility according to what is written in the patient's chart. Medical and legal experts could also scrutinize charts years later should the patient's care result in litigation.

3.2 The Medication Administration Record (MAR)

The Medication Administration Record (MAR) is a working document that lists medications that are ordered for a patient and is used to document whether or not those medications were administered.

The design of a MAR differs among healthcare facilities; however each has the same sections. These are:

Patient Information (Figure 3.1): This includes the patient's name, identification number, room number, diagnosis, and allergies.

Unit	Patient's Name	Allergies		Primary Nurse
Med Surg	Susan Jones	None		Bob Marks
Room #				Social Worker
1601			Age	Roberta Johnson
		52		Resident Physician
			DOB	Dr. Anne Ford
		03/05/59		Attending Physician
				Dr. John Merk

Figure 3.1

Schedule Medications (Figure 3.2): These are medications that are given regularly to the patient to maintain a therapeutic level such as once a day for seven days.

Order Date Initials	Exp. Date Time	Medication-Dosage-Frequency Rt. of Adm.	HR	4/1	4/2	4/3	4/4	4/5	4/6	4/7

Medication Administration Record

Figure 3.2

Single Orders (Figure 3.3): These are medications that are administered once for an immediate effect, such as epinephrine given stat for anaphylactic shock.

Code

O = Omitted	/ = Outdated	Cut = Discontinued
1 = Upper Outer Quadrant R Buttock	7 = Rt. Lateral Thigh	13 = Lt. Anterior Lateral Abdomen
2 = Upper Outer Quadrant L Buttock	8 = Lt. Lateral Thigh	14 = Rt. Posterior Lateral Abdomen
3 = Rt. Deltoid	9 = Rt. Ventrogluteal Area	15 = Lt. Posterior Lateral Abdomen
4 = Lt. Deltoid	10 = Lt. Ventrogluteal Area	16 = Rt. Upper Outer Arm
5 = Rt. Mid Anterior Thigh	11 = Abdomen	17 = Lt. Upper Outer Arm
6 = Lt. Mid Anterior Thigh	12 = Rt. Anterior Lateral Abdomen	

Single Orders—Pre-Operatives Stat Meds

Order Date Initials	Medication-Dosage-Route	Date Time	Adm. Time	Time Given	Site	Nurse Initial

Figure 3.3

PRN (pro re nata) Medications (Figure 3.4): These are medications given *as needed*, such as a nonsteroidal anti-inflammatory drug (NSAID) for pain relief.

PRN Medications								
Order Date Initials	Stop Date	Medication-Dosage-Frequency Rt. of Adm.	PRN Medications—Doses Given					
			Date					
			Time					
			Init.					
			Site					
			Date					
			Time					
			Init.					
			Site					
			Date					
			Time					
			Init.					
			Site					

Figure 3.4

Signature (Figure 3.5): Each practitioner who administers a medication to the patient must be identified by full signature, title, and initials entered into the signature section of the MAR. Initials are then placed on the MAR alongside the medications that the practitioner administered to the patient.

Full Signature	Title	Initial
Bob Marks	RN	BM
Mary Adams	RN	MA

Figure 3.5

3.2.1 Creating a New MAR

A new MAR is created when the patient is admitted to the healthcare facility by the admissions staff or by the unit secretary who enters general information about the patient on the MAR and places it into the Medication Administration Record section of the patient's chart.

Prescriptions, written by a practitioner for medication, are copied from the Medical Orders section of the patient's chart and entered into the appropriate section of the MAR using a process called taking off orders (see Taking Off Orders).

A licensed registered nurse (RN) or a licensed practical nurse (LPN) is responsible for taking off orders, although some healthcare facilities permit the unit secretary to take off orders if reviewed and signed off by the patient's primary nurse. The patient's primary nurse is legally responsible for the accuracy in the transcribing of medical orders on the MAR.

3.2.2   Information About Medications

The MAR is a time-saving tool because it contains information needed to administer medications to a patient except for orders that are cancelled or have not been taken off as yet. It is for this reason that you must always review the latest medical orders prior to administering any medication.

For each medication, the MAR contains:

- *Order Date*: the date that the practitioner ordered the medication

- *Expiration Date*: the date on or after that the order is no longer valid

- *Medication Name*: usually the brand name of the medication

- *Dose*: the amount of the medication the patient receives in a specified period of time

- *Frequency*: the number of doses the patient receives

- *Route of Administration*: the route in which the medication is given to the patient

- *Site of Administration*: site where the medication was administered if medication was an injection

- *Date and Time*: day and hour that the medication must be administered

3.2.3   Using the MAR

At the beginning of each shift, the primary nurse reviews the MAR and identifies medications scheduled to be administered to the patient during the shift. The primary nurse also reviews the patient's chart for any new orders or cancelled orders that were written since the MAR was last updated. These orders, if they exist, are then taken off by the primary nurse.

The nurse makes a note of orders that are scheduled to expire at the end of the shift. Depending on the patient's condition and the nature of the order, the nurse may want to ask the practitioner if the order should be renewed.

Next, each medication is located on the unit. Medications delivered regularly by the pharmacy are usually placed in the patient's drawer in the medical cabinet or in the medication room. Each is labeled with the patient's name, identification, and room number. It is important to locate medications at the beginning of the shift, thus allowing time to follow up with the pharmacy if the medication can't be found.

Before preparing to administer medication, the nurse makes one last check of the Medical Order section of the patient's chart to determine if the practitioner cancelled the order or prescribed new medication. This is an important step since in a busy unit the primary nurse may not have the opportunity to speak directly with the practitioner.

The MAR is updated once the medication is administered to the patient. Some healthcare facilities require the primary nurse to take the MAR into the patient's room when administering medication so the MAR can be immediately updated, giving little room for error.

Other healthcare facilities require the primary nurse to update the MAR immediately upon returning to the nurses' station after administering the medication to the patient. This allows room for error since the primary nurse can easily be distracted and may fail to remember to update the MAR.

The MAR is updated using one of three methods depending on the order:

- *Scheduled medication*: The healthcare provider writes his or her initials in the cells that corresponds to the date and time that the medication was ordered.

- *Single orders*: The healthcare provider writes the date, time, site, and his or her initials.

- *PRN*: The nurse enters the date, time, site, and his or her initials.

Never update the MAR before administering medication.

3.2.4 The Prescription

A prescription is an order for medication that is written on a prescription form if the patient is going to receive it after leaving the healthcare facility.

The practitioner must clearly specify in a prescription the medication and how the medication is to be administered. The prescription must contain the

- Name of the medication
- Dose
- Number of doses
- Route
- Frequency
- Start and end dates for administering

The actual time that the medication is administered is determined by the nurse when pulling down the order, unless the practitioner specifies otherwise. For example, the practitioner may order that the medication be administered twice a day. The nurse determines this means 8 a.m. and 8 p.m. based on the healthcare facility's policy.

The practitioner's medication order may specify a condition must exist before the medication is given to the patient. For example, it is common for a practitioner to order different doses of insulin, called a sliding scale, based on the patient's serum glucose level. The nurse tests the patient's serum glucose and based on the results administers the desired number of units of insulin.

Some healthcare facilities place orders for insulin given on a sliding scale in the Medical Orders section of the patient's chart instead of the prescription section of the MAR.

For a patient being discharged, a prescription is written on a prescription form and placed into the Discharge section of the patient's chart. The nurse then gives the patient the prescription as part of the patient's discharge orders.

3.3 The Kardex

The Kardex is a quick-reference document commonly used on a unit to provide the healthcare team with information about the patient brought together into one place and readily available without having to search through the patient's chart.

Each healthcare facility has its own form of a Kardex. With the integration of a computer charting system, many facilities now have the capability of generating a computer-based Kardex, although some still use cards stored in a flip chart or standard sheets of paper that are stored in a loose-leaf binder. Regardless of the form, all contain the same kind of information.

Information found on a Kardex includes:

Orders for diagnostic procedures and/or treatments (other than medications) (Figure 3.6): These are orders taken off the Medical Order section of the patient's chart for lab tests and procedures used to diagnose the patient. Each is listed along with the date it was ordered (a paper Kardex may indicate the date it was completed). Note, however, that the computer-generated Kardex is printed every day and updated with current orders only—listing as above; information regarding completion of the procedure or treatment would be handed off during a verbal, taped, or written "hand-off" report at the end of every shift.

- *General Patient Information*: This includes patient's name, room number, age, date of birth, allergies, and diagnosis.

- *The Healthcare Team*: The attending practitioner is listed here. On a paper Kardex, other departments involved with the care may be listed; for example, physical therapy, occupational therapy, respiratory therapy. A computer-generated Kardex may only list the attending practitioner; other departments will document involvement with care on the interdisciplinary progress record.

- *Specialty Information*: The medical team caring for patients on a specialty unit such as ICU, psychiatry, and cardiology need key information that otherwise would not be found on a general-purpose Kardex. Therefore, healthcare facilities typically design specialty Kardexes for these units.

Patient Kardex					
Date Ordered	Diagnostic Procedures	Date Done	Date Ordered	Vital Signs/Treatments	Expir. Date

Figure 3.6

3.4   Taking Off Orders

Medical orders written for medication, treatments, and diagnostic tests must be copied from the Medical Orders section of the patient's chart to the MAR and Kardex. This process is called taking off orders. This is a critical process because failure to accurately transfer the order can have serious consequences for the patient.

Many healthcare facilities require an RN to take off orders; however some healthcare facilities authorize trained staff such as an LPN or unit secretary to take off orders if reviewed and signed off by an RN.

Orders for medication contain most, but not all, the information that must be entered into a MAR. Practitioners typically don't specify the exact time to administer scheduled medication. Instead practitioners use medical abbreviations to indicate the number of doses to administer to the patient. For example, the practitioner will write "daily" on the prescription if the patient is to receive one dose per day.

The primary nurse is responsible for translating this into a medication schedule when taking off the order using the healthcare facility's policy as a guide. Some healthcare facilities require that medication ordered once a day be given at 10 a.m.

Orders for treatments and tests also typically lack specific times. The practitioner will write "upper GI series" and the test schedule with other departments in the healthcare facility and then update the Kardex.

3.4.1   How to Take Off an Order

Let's say that the practitioner wrote the following prescription:

Lasix 40 mg PO daily
KCl 20 mEq PO daily

The medications above are considered to be scheduled medications as they indicate that the patient will take them every day until the order expiration date, which is generally seven days after the initial order is written.

In manual systems, the healthcare provider writes the order and flags the chart. This alerts the unit secretary that there is a new order written for the patient. In a computerized system, the order is directly entered into the computerized chart, and the RN electronically signs off on the order.

The primary RN or the charge RN designee verifies the order for its accuracy in the computer. This verification is then seen by the pharmacist who will also verify the order, mark it as a verified order, fill it, and send the medication to the unit for the patient.

In a paper system, the same steps would be taken, and the verification by the RN is noted with his or her initials. A copy is sent to the pharmacy, and the pharmacist will verify the order, fill it, and send it back to the unit.

The nurse then takes off the order by writing it in the MAR as shown in Figure 3.7.

Medication Administration Record

Order Date Initials	Exp. Date Time	Medication-Dosage-Frequency Rt. of Adm.	HR	4/1	4/2	4/3	4/4	4/5	4/6	4/7
4/1 BM	4/7	Ativan 60 mg PO q.i.d.	00:00							
			06:00							
			12:00							
			18:00							

Figure 3.7

The practitioner might write a single order for medication such as:

Morphine sulfate 2 mg IVP now × 1

In a single order the nurse can follow that order only once and the order expires. In a computer system, the nurse will enter the order, administer the medication, and chart it as given. The unit secretary can also enter this order, and then the system as above will follow for RN/pharmacist verification. In a paper system, the medication is written in the designated area for one-time-only medications and the system above is followed. This is illustrated in Figure 3.8.

Code

O = Omitted	/ = Outdated	Cut = Discontinued
1 = Upper Outer Quadrant R Buttock	7 = Rt. Lateral Thigh	13 = Lt. Anterior Lateral Abdomen
2 = Upper Outer Quadrant L Buttock	8 = Lt. Lateral Thigh	14 = Rt. Posterior Lateral Abdomen
3 = Rt. Deltoid	9 = Rt. Ventrogluteal Area	15 = Lt. Posterior Lateral Abdomen
4 = Lt. Deltoid	10 = Lt. Ventrogluteal Area	16 = Rt. Upper Outer Arm
5 = Rt. Mid Anterior Thigh	11 = Abdomen	17 = Lt. Upper Outer Arm
6 = Lt. Mid Anterior Thigh	12 = Rt. Anterior Lateral Abdomen	

Single Orders—Pre-Operatives Stat Meds

Order Date Initials	Medication-Dosage-Route	Date Time	Adm. Time	Time Given	Site	Nurse Initial
12/1/13 JK	Ativan 2 mg 1 time	12/1/13 17:00	17:00	17:00	3	JK

Figure 3.8

PRN is another type of prescription that the practitioner might write as:

Zofran 4 mg IVP q6h PRN for nausea
Acetaminophen 650 mg PO q6h PRN for temp >100.5

The system in place for taking off a PRN order would be the same as the system used for a one time order and/or a scheduled medication. PRN orders are placed in the PRN area of the MAR as shown in Figure 3.9.

PRN Medications								
Order Date Initials	**Stop Date**	**Medication-Dosage-Frequency Rt. of Adm.**	**PRN Medications—Doses Given**					
4/1	4/7	*Haldol 5 mg PO q4h*	Date	4/1				
			Time	08:00				
BM			Init.	BM				
			Site					
			Date					
			Time					
			Init.					
			Site					
			Date					
			Time					
			Init.					
			Site					

Figure 3.9

Treatment orders must also be taken off and placed in the Kardex. Say that the practitioner ordered the following treatment and two medical tests:

Nebulizer Albuterol (2.5 mg/3mL) 2.5 mg/Ipratropium (0.5/2.5 mg) 0.5 mg q4 & q2 PRN for audible wheezing
MRI Brain with contrast, Indications: R/O meningitis
MRI ABD without contrast, organ to be scanned, Indications: R/O biliary mass

Treatment orders and medical orders are both handled the same way, and similar to any medication order, following the system check between unit secretary and RN. Once the orders are verified, they will appear on a computer-generated Kardex with the date of order; they will appear on a paper Kardex with a date of order and a date of completion when appropriate. This is shown in Figure 3.10.

Patient Kardex						
Date Ordered	**Diagnostic Procedures**	**Date Done**	**Date Ordered**	**Vital Signs/Treatments**	**Expir. Date**	
1/4/13	*Chest X-Ray r/o abnormalities*	1/4/13	1/3/13	*BP 132/88 P76 R18 Reg 98 T*	1/3/13	
1/6/13	*CT Scan ABN w/o contrast r/o*	1/7/13				
	abnormalities					

Figure 3.10

3.5 Avoid Common Errors When Using MAR and Kardex

Errors can occur when taking off orders and recording when medication is administered to a patient resulting in overmedicating or under medicating the patient or administering incorrect medication.

Steps can be taken to assure that the most common of these errors is avoided. Here are some steps to take:

Use abbreviations that are approved by the Joint Commission and adopted by your healthcare facility. For example, all healthcare facilities require that "daily" replace the abbreviation OD and "every other day" be used in place of QOD. Always write the full word if you are unsure of the abbreviation to write. Refer to your facility's "dangerous abbreviations" policy for clarification.

The Joint Commission requires writing numbers by dropping the zero following a decimal if the dose is a whole number and use a zero to the left of the decimal if the dose is a fraction. Write 1 mg instead of 1.0 mg and 0.5 mg instead of .5 mg.

The healthcare provider should be sure that his or her full name, title, and initials appear on the MAR and KARDEX before initializing that a medication was administered or a procedure or diagnostic test was performed.

Update the MAR immediately after the medication is administered to the patient.

Write legibly on all documents. Assume all handwriting is difficult to read and make certain all entries are legible.

Circle any medication that wasn't administered and write the reason why it was omitted in the MAR or in the nurse progress notes if there isn't sufficient space to include comments in the MAR. (Check your healthcare facility's policy for further instruction.)

Write in the MAR the reason for administering PRN medication.

Note the assessment results on the MAR if particular assessments must be made before administering medication (i.e., the patient's blood pressure before administering blood pressure medication).

If the patient refuses medication, write the patient's own words in quotations in the MAR and/or in the nurse progress notes and other documents required by your healthcare facility.

3.6 Charting Narcotics

Healthcare facilities require additional documentation for opioids. Many healthcare facilities use a computer-controlled cabinet (Pyxis) located in the medication room to dispense opioids. The computer automatically documents dispensing the medication, which includes the medication, dose, patient, and the nurse who retrieved the medication.

Healthcare facilities that don't use a computer-controlled cabinet manually document the inventory of opioids within the locked area of the medication room by using the opioids inventory control form.

At the beginning of each shift, one RN from the offgoing shift and an RN from the oncoming shift count the number of opioids in the medication room and compare the total to the current balance on the opioids inventory control form. Any difference is reported to the nursing supervisor.

During the shift the patient's primary nurse records the name, dose, and patient's identifier on the opioids inventory control form and signs the form when preparing to administer the opioid to a patient. This amount is deducted from the current balance and a new balance is entered on the opioids inventory control form.

Any opioid that is discarded must be witnessed by a nurse. Both the primary nurse and the witness must sign the opioids inventory control form stating the reason for discarding the medication.

3.7 IV Administration

IV medications are documented on an IV administration form that is sometimes combined with a fluid intake and output form (Figure 3.11). Additional information is entered into the nurse progress notes. Every aspect of administering the IV should be documented.

IV Administration				
Time	IV Fluid/Blood Products	Rate	CC's Hung/LIB	Condition
00:00				
01:00				
02:00				
03:00				
04:00				
05:00				
06:00				
07:00				
Total				
08:00				
09:00				
10:00				
11:00				
12:00				
13:00				
14:00				
15:00				
Total				
16:00				
17:00				
18:00				
19:00				
20:00				
21:00				
22:00				
23:00				
Total				

Figure 3.11

Here is the information that the healthcare provider needs to include:

- Date and time administration began

- Name of medication or blood product given to the patient

- Type and location of the IV lock

- Complications such as number of attempts to insert the lock and who inserted the lock

- The amount of IV fluid hung

- The rate of flow of the IV

- Whether or not a gravity feed or a pump is used

At least each shift, it is necessary to examine the IV site and assess the IV flow. The healthcare provider needs to document:

- The condition of the IV site (see Figure 3.11)

- The flushing of the lock with saline or heparin solution

- The date, time, and the amount of fluid left in the bag if the IV is stopped and removed

- The amount of fluid left in the bag if it is changed and the amount of fluid and rate of flow if a new bag is hung

- The date, time, type, and location of the IV lock if the location of the IV lock was changed

3.8   Intake and Output Flow Chart

It is important for a practitioner to know the amount of fluids a patient receives and the amount of fluids that the patient excretes in a 24-hour period depending on the nature of the patient's condition. This is commonly referred to as the patient's intake and output and is recorded on the Intake and Output form (Figures 3.12 and 3.13).

INTAKE				
IV CC's Rec'd	PO	Tube Feed	NG/GI IRRIG.	Hourly Running Total
Total Intake, 24 HRS:				

Figure 3.12

Intake includes liquids that the patient

- Takes by mouth (meals)
- Through gastrostomy (PEG) feeding tubes
- Through nasogastric (NG) feeding tubes
- IV fluids
- Blood or its components
- Liquid medication
- Fluids used to flush tubes

Output includes:

- Urine
- Diarrhea

- Vomitus
- Gastric suction
- Wound drainage and type of drain

Time	NG/GI	STOOL	MESIS	URINE	OTHER	Hourly Running Total
|	**Output**					
00:00						
01:00						
02:00						
03:00						
04:00						
05:00						
06:00						
07:00						
Total						
08:00						
09:00						
10:00						
11:00						
12:00						
13:00						
14:00						
15:00						
Total						
16:00						
17:00						
18:00						
19:00						
20:00						
21:00						
22:00						
23:00						
Total						
				Total Output, 24 HRS:		

Figure 3.13

The amount of fluid is entered in the appropriate cell in the Input and Output form according to the time and nature of the fluid. It is important to record fluids in milliliters, although some healthcare facilities might use centimeters as the unit of measurement. This means that the healthcare provider will need to convert household measurements to milliliters (ml) before recording it (Table 3.1).

TABLE 3.1 **Converting Common Household Measurements**

HOUSEHOLD MEASUREMENT	MILLILITER EQUIVALENT
1 ounce	30 ml
1 teaspoon	5 ml
1 tablespoon	15 ml

Most fluid taken by the patient is premeasured, making it straightforward to record the volume on the Intake and Output form. Likewise, most fluid excreted by the patient can be easily measured using an appropriate device. However, it will be necessary to measure fluid intake and output that isn't premeasured or is difficult to measure.

For example, ice chips would be written as ice chips or approximated as sips—10 ml and so forth; Jell-O or gelatin is measured by milliliters—an approximate amount based on the container size of the product.

3.8.1 Avoiding Common Mistakes

Here are common errors that occur when measuring intake and output. Knowing these will help the healthcare provider to avoid them.

Intake

- The patient eats snacks and drinks juice or soft drinks without the knowledge of the nurse.
- IV push medication is not included.
- IV piggybacks are not recorded.
- The flushing of tubes is not recorded.
- Fluids are taken while the patient undergoes tests outside of the unit.
- Fluids such as liquid medication are swallowed.

Output

- The patient who has bathroom privileges voids and fails to notify the nurse.
- Bleeding is not recorded.
- Incontinence is not taken into account.

3.9 Transferring a Patient

Every time a patient is moved from one unit to another the transfer must be documented in the nurse's notes. The nurse's notes contain pertinent information that describes the transfer for both the current unit and the receiving unit.

Some healthcare facilities use a special document called a trip ticket. A trip ticket is used when the patient is leaving with a transporter or unlicensed person. The trip ticket indicates where the patient is going and why he or she is going off the unit.

The trip ticket contains general information such as:

- Date and time of the transfer
- Name of the current unit
- Name of the receiving unit

The nurse's notes also describe the condition of the patient when the patient left the unit and the condition of the patient when the patient arrived at the new unit. The reason for the transfer is also documented. Any change in the patient's condition that occurs during the transfer is noted.

Be sure to include:

- Description of any wounds
- Location of heparin locks

- Description of medical devices that are connected to the patient during the transfer

- Vital signs

- Allergies

- Advance directives

- Significant procedures or events involving the patient

- The patient's ability to communicate

- Names of staff who accompanied the patient during the transfer

3.9.1 Documenting a Transfer

The nurse must assess the patient before the patient is transferred and document this assessment in the nurse's notes. Only a stable patient should leave the unit with an unlicensed person.

An unstable patient should not be transferred unless the patient is accompanied by an RN and is monitored constantly with an electrocardiogram or other appropriate equipment. This should be noted in the nurse's notes.

The patency of oxygen, IV, and other forms of ongoing treatment must be assessed and noted in the nurse's notes before the patient leaves the unit.

As a precaution the transfer RN needs to assess the patient prior to transfer.

3.9.2 Giving a Charge Report

The nurse who is taking over primary care for the patient in the receiving unit must be brought up-to-date on the patient's status. This is accomplished when the patient's current primary nurse gives the charge report.

The charge report is verbal documentation of the patient's condition. It can be given over the telephone before the patient arrives on the unit or in person if the primary nurse accompanies the patient to the new unit.

The transfer of a patient isn't complete until the charge report is given to the nurse who is accepting primary care for the patient. The charge report should follow the Joint Commission standards for hand-off communications. This standard is easy to follow by remembering the acronym ISBAR.

Here is the information that should be provided to the other nurse:

- *Introduction*: The nurse identifies himself or herself and the patient.

- *Situation*: The nurse tells the new nurse the patient's chief complaint and/or diagnosis, including significant events and the patient's needs and problems.

- *Background*: The nurse gives a synopsis of the patient's treatment, vital signs, pain level, complaints, and assessment changes.

- *Assessment*: The nurse provides the new nurse with a conclusion about the patient's situation, overall body systems involved, and if the patient is in a life-threatening situation.

- *Recommendation*: The nurse tells the new nurse any information that would be helpful, such as medications and tests scheduled for the patient, if the patient will be transferred again, and a clarification of all orders.

Another acronym that is handy to remember when giving a transfer or end-of-shift report is I-PASS-THE-BATON.

- *Introduction*: The nurse introduces himself.

- *Patient*: The patient is identified.

- *Assessment*: Chief complaint and/or diagnosis, vital signs, and symptoms are provided.

- *Situation*: Code status, circumstances, recent changes, response to treatment, and current status are given.

- *Safety concerns*: Critical labs, reports, allergies, alerts (falls, isolation, and so forth) are noted.

- *Background*: Comorbidities, family history, current medications, and previous episodes are provided.

- *Actions*: The nurse indicates what actions have been taken or required and what the rationale for the action is.

- *Timing*: Level of urgency and prioritization of actions are identified.

- *Ownership*: Who is responsible? Nurse/doctor/team? Patient/patient family?

- *Next*: What will happen next? Plans? Anticipated changes?

Solved Problems

3.1   What is a MAR?

The Medication Administration Record (MAR) is a working document that lists medications that are ordered for a patient and is used to document whether or not those medications were administered.

3.2   What is the Schedule Medications section of a MAR?

These are medications that are given regularly to the patient to maintain a therapeutic level, such as once a day for seven days.

3.3   What is the Single Orders section of a MAR?

These are medications that are administered once for an immediate effect, such as epinephrine given stat for anaphylactic shock.

3.4   What is the PRN Medications section of a MAR?

These are medications given as needed, such as a nonsteroidal anti-inflammatory drug (NSAID) for pain relief.

3.5   What is the signature section of the MAR?

Each practitioner who administers a medication to the patient must be identified by full signature, title, and initials entered into the signature section of the MAR. Initials are then placed on the MAR alongside the medications that the practitioner administered to the patient.

3.6   When is a MAR created?

A new MAR is created when the patient is admitted to the healthcare facility by the admissions staff or by the unit secretary who enters general information about the patient on the MAR and places it into the Medication Administration Record section of the patient's chart.

3.7   What is contained in a MAR?

- Order Date: This is the date that the practitioner ordered the medication.

- Expiration Date: The order is no longer valid on or after the expiration date of the order.

- Medication Name: This is usually the brand name of the medication.

- Dose: This is the amount of the medication the patient receives in a specified period of time.

- Frequency: This is the number of doses the patient receives.

- Route of Administration: This is the route in which the medication is given to the patient.

- Site of Administration: If the medication was administered as an injection, this indicates the site of the injection.

- Date and Time: This is the day and hour that the medication must be administered.

3.8   What are the three methods used to update a MAR?

- Scheduled medication: The healthcare provider writes her initials in the cells that corresponds to the date and time that the medication was ordered.

- Single orders: The healthcare provider writes the date, time, and site and initials this.

- PRN: The date, time, and site are entered and initialed.

3.9   What is a prescription?

A prescription is an order for medication that is written on a prescription form if the patient is going to receive it after leaving the healthcare facility.

3.10   What information must be contained on a prescription?

- Name of the medication

- Dose

- Number of doses

- Route

- Frequency

- Start and end dates for administering

3.11   What is the best defense against malpractice action?

The best defense against a malpractice suit is accurately documenting patient care.

3.12   How does a practitioner specify when a PRN is given?

The practitioner's medication order may specify a condition must exist before the medication is given to the patient.

3.13   What is a Kardex?

The Kardex is a quick reference document commonly used on a unit to provide the healthcare team with information about the patient brought together in one place and readily available without having to search through the patient's chart.

3.14   What kind of information is contained in the Kardex?

- Orders for diagnostic procedures and/or treatments other than medications

- General patient information

- The healthcare team

- Specialty information

3.15   What is taking off orders?

Medical orders written for medication, treatments, and diagnostic tests must be copied from the Medical Orders section of the patient's chart to the MAR and Kardex. This process is called taking off orders.

3.16   Who can take off orders?

Many healthcare facilities require an RN to take off orders; however some healthcare facilities authorize trained staff such as an LPN or unit secretary to take off orders if reviewed and signed off by an RN.

3.17   How are orders written?

In manual systems, the healthcare provider writes the order and flags the chart. This alerts the unit secretary that there is a new order written for the patient. In a computerized system, the order is entered directly into the computerized chart and the RN electronically signs off on the order.

3.18   What is a single order?

In a single order the nurse can follow that order only once and the order expires.

3.19   What medical abbreviations should be used in charting?

Use abbreviations that are approved by the Joint Commission and adopted by your healthcare facility.

3.20   What should the nurse do when he sees "OD" used?

Remind the practitioner that "daily" should be used in place of OD. OD is not an approved medical abbreviation.

3.21   How should decimal values be written?

The Joint Commission requires writing numbers by dropping the zero following a decimal if the dose is a whole number and use a zero to the left of the decimal if the dose is a fraction. Write 1 mg instead of 1.0 mg and 0.5 mg instead of .5 mg.

3.22   What should be documented when administering a PRN medication?

Write in the MAR the reason for administering a PRN medication.

3.23   What should be documented for IV administration?

- Date and time administration began

- Name of medication or blood product given to the patient

- Type and location of the IV lock

- Complications such as number of attempts to insert the lock and who inserted the lock

- The amount of IV fluid hung

- The rate of flow of the IV

- Whether or not gravity feed or a pump is used

3.24   What must be performed and documented each shift when a patient is receiving an IV?

- The condition of the IV site (see Figure 3.11)

- Flushing the lock with saline or heparin solution

- The date, time, and the amount of fluid left in the bag if the IV is stopped and removed

- The amount of fluid left in the bag if the bag is changed and the amount of fluid and rate of flow if a new bag is hung

- The date, time, type, and location of the IV lock if the location of the IV lock is changed

3.25   What should be documented as fluid outflow?

- Urine

- Diarrhea

- Vomitus

- Gastric suction

- Wound drainage and type of drain

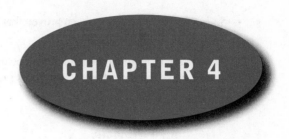

CHAPTER 4

Patient Care Plans

4.1 Definition

The patient's healthcare team works from an interdisciplinary patient care plan used to guide the healthcare team through diagnostic tests, medical procedures, and routines that assure that the patient receives the best possible care. There are many forms of care plans, all of which contain the same key information to direct the healthcare team.

- The patient's problem(s)
- Interventions to address each problem
- The expected outcome or goal of these interventions
- Evaluation of the intervention

4.2 Care Plan Objective

A care plan contains the patient's healthcare problems that were identified when the patient was assessed, and it contains actions for the healthcare team to take to minimize or resolve those problems. The action is a work plan, and the healthcare team can measure the results to learn if the action did minimize or resolve the patient's problem. Each action:

- Must be based on a scientific rationale
- Have a measurable outcome
- Be patient specific

For example:

- *Problem*: A patient on total bed rest is at risk for decubitus ulcers (bedsores).
- *Action*: The healthcare team will turn the position of the patient in bed every two hours.

- *Scientific Rationale*: It has been proven that turning the position of the patient frequently will reduce the risk for decubitus ulcers.

- *Evaluation*: Examining the patient for decubitus ulcers at the beginning of each shift determines if repositioning the patient every two hours prevented decubitus ulcers.

4.2.1 Defining a Problem

Assessment of the patient's signs and symptoms enables the healthcare team to define the patient's problem(s). Each problem is described as a nursing diagnosis. A nursing diagnosis is a standardized statement defined by a recognized body such as the North American Nursing Diagnosis Association (NANDA). The problem is described in the nursing plan using the nursing diagnosis.

There are many styles of care plans. Some care plans will use the PES format to identify a problem. The PES format has three components:

- **P** is the problem identified by the nursing diagnosis

- **E** is the etiology-origin of the problem

- **S** is the signs or symptoms that lead the healthcare team to choose this nursing diagnosis

The PES format is written as:

- P: nursing diagnosis from the NANDA list of nursing diagnosis

- E: related to (specify the patient's medical condition)

- S: as evidence by (list signs and symptoms)

For example, a patient who is being treated for deep tissue laceration of the left inferior calf is experiencing pain. Here is one way to describe this problem using the PES format:

- P: acute pain

- E: related to deep tissue laceration of the left inferior calf

- S: as evidenced by the patient reporting a pain level 8 on a scale of 0 to 10

4.2.2 Setting Goals

Goals are set for each patient problem. A goal is a measurable outcome that is expected after the healthcare team performs the action. The number of goals defined depends on the nature of the patient's problem.

Each goal is assessed after the action is performed to determine if the desired result was achieved. The assessment is made using a standard measurement, which many times involves the patient reporting a condition or performing a behavior.

A measurement can be subjective or objective. For example, measuring pain is subjective based on the patient's definition of pain. A temperature of 100°F is objective and is not influenced by interpretation. Both subjective and objective measurements can be used to set goals.

Goals for the patient with a deep tissue laceration are:

1. Patient will report an acceptable pain level on a scale of 0 to 10.

2. Patient will report that the pain management regimen relieves pain to satisfactory level with acceptable and manageable side effects.

3. Patient will perform activities of recovery with reported acceptable level of pain.

4.2.3   Planning Action

An action is something done to achieve goals that were set for the patient with regard to the nursing diagnosis. Actions are related to goals. Each goal could have one or more actions. An action can achieve one or more goals depending on the goal and the action.

Each action begins with a verb such as "assess," "assist," "explain," and "teach" and is followed by the description of the action. Here are a few actions for the patient with a deep tissue laceration.

1. Assess the patient's pain level every 2 hours and PRN (as needed) using the scale of 0 to 10.

2. Teach the patient to use stabilizing equipment or supportive measures when moving.

3. Assist the patient with ADLs (activities of daily living—e.g., use of bedpan) as needed to manage pain level.

4. Teach the patient the myths and facts regarding physical and psychological addiction to narcotics.

5. Teach the patient to request pain medication before pain is severe.

4.2.4   Scientific Rationale

There must be a scientific basis for each action. The scientific basis is a recognized standard of practice that is documented in a healthcare facilities policy or by an authoritative source.

An institutional care plan will not include a scientific rationale for interventions. Student care plans will specify a scientific rationale. Healthcare facilities standardize care plans according to patient profiles. Goals, actions, and other components of the care plan are predefined based on scientific rationale and can be modified as needed to address the needs of the patient.

The scientific rationale is a sentence or paragraph that justifies the action followed by a reference. Rationales are numbered according to the number of the corresponding action.

Here are scientific rationales for actions for the patient with a deep tissue laceration:

1. The patient's verbalization of pain on a scale of 0 to 10 determines the effectiveness of pain medication administered to the patient. (Paulette D. Rollant and Deborah A. Ennis, *Mosby's Medical-Surgical Nursing* [Maryland Heights: Mosby, 2001], p. 138, ISBN–10: 0323011772)

2. Supporting an injured leg reduces pressure on the wound and reduces pain to the patient. (Patricia A. Potter and Anne Griffin Perry, *Fundamentals of Nursing* [Maryland Heights: Mosby, 2007], p. 1483, ISBN–10: 0323054234)

3. Positioning a bedpan can be extremely uncomfortable. The nurse should help position the patient comfortably and support wound areas. (Patricia A. Potter and Anne Griffin Perry, *Fundamentals of Nursing* [Maryland Heights: Mosby, 2007], p. 1395, ISBN–10: 0323054234)

4. The patient may withhold self-medication for fear of developing addiction to pain medication. (Paulette D. Rollant and Deborah A. Ennis, *Mosby's Medical-Surgical Nursing* [Maryland Heights: Mosby, 2001], p. 154, ISBN–10: 0323011772)

5. Treatment for pain requires that pain medication be given before pain occurs. (Paulette D. Rollant and Deborah A. Ennis, *Mosby's Medical-Surgical Nursing* [Maryland Heights: Mosby, 2001], p. 140, ISBN–10: 0323011772)

4.2.5   Evaluating the Outcome

The outcome of every action is evaluated to determine if the action impacted the patient and whether or not the goal was achieved. The outcome is described in a sentence or paragraph that usually begins with *the patient* followed by an explanation of how the patient reacted to the action and if the goal associated with the action was reached.

Goals are not always 100 percent achieved. The level of achievement is indicated in the evaluation. An outcome may not be observed for a number of reasons. In these cases, write "not observed."

Each evaluation is numbered to correspond with the goal. Here are evaluations for the patient with a deep tissue laceration:

1. The patient reported a pain level of 8 on a scale of 0 to 10 when moving his left calf 20 minutes after the pain medication dose peaked.

2. The patient demonstrated correct use of the leg immobilizer prior to moving self out of bed.

3. The patient called the nurse for assistance when using the bedpan.

4. Patient verbalized that requesting pain medication frequently will not lead to addiction.

5. Patient successfully anticipated pain and used the call button to ask the nurse for PRN medication. He frequently reports a pain level of 2 on a scale of 0 to 10.

4.3   Categories of Nursing Diagnosis

There are five categories of nursing diagnosis (NANDA). Each category contains a nursing diagnosis that can easily be mapped to the condition of the patient. The categories are:

- Actual Diagnosis focuses on the patient's health problem such as acute pain.

- Risk Diagnosis consists of potential problems that the patient is at risk for developing and begins with *risk for*, such as *risk for injury*.

- Possible Diagnosis consists of problems that the patient may have, but there is insufficient information to make the diagnosis. This begins with *possible*, such as *possible fluid volume excess*.

- Syndrome Diagnosis is a problem that consists of a cluster of other diagnoses such as chronic pain.

- Wellness Diagnosis consists of problems that could arise because of the patient's ill health and usually begins with, for example, *potential for*.

4.4   Care Plan Formats

All care plan formats serve as a guide for providing care to the patient. Each care plan format differs in the format style and the kind of information contained in the care plan.

Two care plan formats commonly used are:

- *Nursing care plan*: A comprehensive style required by nursing schools.

- *Interdisciplinary care plan (care map)*: A comprehensive, interdisciplinary plan that identifies care over a 24-hour period delivered by all members of the patient's healthcare team.

4.4.1 Nursing Care Plan

The nursing care plan typically consists of six columns, although this will vary from school to school. Keep in mind, however, that prior to the columns, the school's care plan has asked the student to provide a comprehensive assessment and has provided the student with space for this. The assessment section in a student care plan will reflect the same information that a nurse would find in an institutional chart. This consists of:

- Admission database
- History and physical, including current and past medical and surgical history and results of the most current physical examination findings
- Social history
- Laboratory results data
- Diagnostic data
- Medication history

The first column is typically the assessment column for the identified problem. This column reflects the supporting data or the defining characteristics that lead you to the formation of the nursing diagnosis or the patient's problem (stating one problem at a time).

The assessment data or defining characteristics for the diagnosis or problem of pain might include information such as pain level, medications ordered for treatment, and statements made by the patient that describe the pain level (Figure 4.1).

ASSESSMENT
(Defining Characteristics—Supporting Data)

- Pain level 8/10
- Using PCA Morphine pump
  continually
- Grimaces with any movement
- States "Pain is unbearable"

Figure 4.1

The next two columns (Figure 4.2) define the patient's problem (see Defining a Problem) and setting goals for the treatment (see Setting Goals). These columns are followed by three additional columns (Figure 4.3) that specify planning (see Planning Action), scientific rationales (see Scientific Rationale), and evaluating the intervention (see Evaluating the Outcome) taken by the medical team to address the patient's problem.

DIAGNOSIS	GOALS
Problem, Etiology, Symptoms P: Acute pain E: Related to deep tissue laceration left inferior calf S: As evidence by the patient reporting a pain level of 8 on a scale of 0 to 10	Patient will report an acceptable pain level on a scale of 0 to 10. Patient will report that pain management regimen relieves pain to satisfactory level with acceptable and manageable side effects. Patient will perform activities of recovery with reported acceptable level of pain.

Figure 4.2

PLANNING INTERVENTIONS	SCIENTIFIC RATIONALES	EVALUATION
1. Assess the patient's pain level every two hours and PRN using the scale of 0 to 10.	1. The patient's verbalization of pain on a scale of 0 to 10 determines the effectiveness of pain medication administered to the patient (Mosby, *Medical-Surgical Nursing*, p. 138).	1. The patient reported a pain level of 8 on a scale of 0 to 10 when moving left calf 20 minutes after the pain medication dose peaked.
2. Teach the patient to use stabilizing equipment or supporting measures when moving.	2. Supporting an injured leg reduces pressure on the wound and reduces pain to the patient (Potter, *Fundamentals of Nursing*, p. 1483).	2. The patient demonstrated correct use of the leg immobilizer prior to moving self out of bed.
3. Assist patient with ADLs to help manage pain level.	3. Positioning a bedpan can be extremely uncomfortable. The nurse should help position clients comfortably and support wound areas (Potter, *Fundamentals of Nursing*, p. 1395).	3. The patient called the nurse for assistance each time he felt a BM; however he did not have a BM while under the nurse's care.
4. Teach patient myths/facts regarding: physical/psychological addiction to narcotics.	4. The patient may withhold self-medication for fear of developing addiction to pain medication (Mosby, *Medical-Surgical Nursing*, p. 154).	4. Patient verbalized that requesting pain medication frequently will not lead to addiction.
5. Teach patient to request pain medication before pain is severe.	5. Treatment for pain requires that pain medication be given before pain occurs (Mosby, *Medical-Surgical Nursing*, p.140).	5. Patient successfully anticipated pain and used the call button to ask the nurse for PRN medication. He frequently reports a pain level of 2 (0–10).

Figure 4.3

Figure 4.4 suggests another style of care plan where the plan is put together in three columns instead of six. This can resemble some student care plans or may be seen as an institutional care plan part of the care map (see Interdisciplinary Care Plans).

Patient Problem	Expected Outcome	Nursing Orders
Respiratory: Risk for aspiration pneumonia as indicated by a. Pseudobulbar symptoms b. Bedridden	Normal respiration patterns No congestion Afebrile	1. Position the patient upright during feeding 2. Blenderized food 3. Feed the patient small portions 4. Deep breathing and coughing exercise q4h during waking hours

Figure 4.4

4.4.2   Interdisciplinary Care Plans

Interdisciplinary care plans, called care maps, are used by most healthcare institutions to provide continuity of care given by members of the patient's healthcare team to the patient, and also provide a uniformed approach to identifying the patient's needs, treatment, and expected outcomes. The interdisciplinary care plan is initiated by the nurse, and the patient's healthcare team addresses issues on the plan as indicated.

The interdisciplinary care plan is a combination of a care plan and the various documentation/charting tools that the healthcare team uses to document the care. These tools include the admission database and serve as the comprehensive assessment tool for patient care using the nursing process as a foundation.

The format of the care plan portion of the care map may look similar to a student care plan in that it may use a columnar format as shown in Figure 4.4. Regardless of the format, the interdisciplinary care plan is a comprehensive picture of all the patient's problems identified for this hospitalization.

The interdisciplinary care plan is divided into categories of patient care:

- Nutrition

- Assessment and treatment

- Teaching and psychosocial

- Specimens and diagnostics

- Safety and activity

- Discharge plan

Each category contains interventions that are commonly performed by the healthcare team. Alongside each intervention is a box for day, evening, and night shifts to initial after the intervention is performed.

4.4.2.1   Nutrition

The nutrition category (Figure 4.5) contains a description of the patient's diet as one of the standard hospital diets as ordered by the practitioner. Table 4.1 contains diets commonly used in hospitals.

Also listed is the percentage of breakfast, lunch, and dinner consumed by the patient. The percentage is a rough estimate by the patient's primary nurse based on observation and not what the patient reports. The patient may report not eating very much and yet consume 75 percent of his meal.

	D	E	N
Diet: *REG*	AB		
Diet Consumed:			
Breakfast 80%	AB		
Lunch 50%	AB		
Dinner 100%	AB		
Enteral feedings: *50 ml/hr SUSTACAL*	AB		
Parenteral Feedings: TPN/Lipids			
Daily Weight 150 lb.-standing scale			

Figure 4.5

TABLE 4.1 Common Hospital Diets

DIET	DESCRIPTION
Low residue	No fiber, no cellulose
High residue	Fiber, cellulose, cabbage, broccoli, apples, brown breads
Low fat	No saturated fat
Full liquid	All liquids, soft-boiled eggs (this is mechanically soft), custard
Clear liquid	Water, tea, no milk.
Sodium restricted	2000 mg; mild 1500–3000 mg; modest 500–1500 mg; severe 500 mg
Ulcer diet	No tea, no coffee, no raw foods, no hot foods, no cold foods
Gluten-free diet (BROW)	No barley, no rye, no oats, no wheat
Diabetic diet	1200, 1400, 1500, 1600, 2000, or 2200 calories

There is also a subcategory for enteral feedings and parenteral feedings, which are based on medical orders. The nurse will document the type or name of the supplement the patient is receiving based on the medical order and the rate at which the supplement is administered.

The nutrition section has space to include the patient's daily weight recorded at the patient at the same time each day using the same scale and having the patient dressed in the same attire. Weights are often recorded at the end of the night shift by the nursing assistant. Generally, the person charting the weight will indicate somewhere on the document the scale used—standing scale, bed scale, chair scale. It is also allowable to refer to the scale by the brand or company name. Weights will be documented either by kilograms or pounds, according to the hospital policy.

4.4.2.2 Assessment and Treatment

An interdisciplinary care plan has a section (Figure 4.6) that identifies standard assessments and treatment that most patients are expected to receive while admitted to a unit. Assessment and treatment reflect the specialty of the unit.

	D	E	N
Cardiac Monitor	AB		
Vital signs q __ 4_ hrs	AB		
I & O q __ 8_ hrs	AB		
D/C Foley			
O2 Therapy: 3 LITERS NC	AB		
O2 Sat q __8_ hrs	AB		
Incentive spirometry q 1 hr. while awake	AB		
C&DB q 1 hr. while awake	AB		
IV fluids as ordered. D/C IV _____ change to PIID	AB		
Dressing change q _ 24__ hrs			
Tubes and drains: Type: _____			
Pain Management PO _____ IM PRN _____ PCA _____ Epidural _____ Continuous IV Infusion _____	AB		
DVT Prophylaxis: Thigh/Knee High TEDS	AB		
Hygiene & Comfort	AB		
Peripheral IV Therapy	AB		
Pressure Ulcer Prevention	AB		
Respiratory Care	AB		

Figure 4.6

Each day, every shift uses the same plan to document the required assessments and treatment. This assures continuity of care among shifts. Each nurse initials the assessment or treatment indicating that it was performed.

Here are the standard assessments and treatments that may be found in a surgical unit:

- Vital signs at an interval specified by the practitioner
- Oxygen therapy at a specified rate and delivery method according to practitioner orders
- Monitoring oxygen saturation at an interval specified by the practitioner

- Administering the incentive spirometry every waking hour

- Cough and deep breath exercises every waking hour

- A description of IV fluids according to medical orders, including the status of the IV site

- Intervals for assessing the site of any wounds and dressing changes

- Identifying drains and assessing the drainage

- Monitoring input and output

- The date a Foley catheter was inserted and the size of the catheter

- The date that the Foley catheter was discontinued

- A description of pain medication and an assessment of its effectiveness

- Orders for treatment that prevent deep vein thrombosis

- Treatment for preventing pressure ulcer

4.4.2.3 Teaching and Psychosocial

The teaching and psychosocial section of an interdisciplinary care plan focuses on the teaching needs of the patient and the family and/or significant others involved in the care. Teaching is the critical part of the discharge plan and begins on the day of admission.

The goal of teaching is to prepare the patient for the discharge from the current level of medical care to home and/or a different level of care. The nurse provides the patient and others with comprehensive information that will facilitate the patient's ability to be cared for once outside the current medical facility.

Each shift, the primary nurse documents any new information given to the patient. The nurse indicates the topic taught, the method used for teaching, any barriers to teaching that may exist, and the patient's response to the teaching.

For example, the nurse may teach the Spanish-speaking patient newly diagnosed with diabetes how to check a blood sugar. Documentation will include the equipment used to teach the skill, the method used to overcome the language barrier, and the patient's ability to demonstrate the skill learned to the nurse.

Most interdisciplinary care plans have a table or key designed to address the criteria; the nurse will also include a narrative note to describe the intervention. The care plan portion of the interdisciplinary care plan will also include the nursing diagnosis (problem) of knowledge deficit. The nurse is expected to teach the patient all aspects of his or her care, thus relieving any anxiety that the patient may have regarding the diagnosis and the discharge plan.

Other examples of topics discussed for teaching include medications (action, frequency, side effects, medication interactions), dressing changes, diet changes, and/or lifestyle changes regarding a new diagnosis. The perioperative nurse is required to teach many aspects of the care including preoperative and postoperative treatments and medications.

4.4.2.4 Specimens and Diagnostics

The Specimens and Diagnostics section (Figure 4.7) lists medical tests and procedures that are ordered by the practitioner. Each entry contains the test or procedure name, the date that the test or procedure should be performed, and whether or not the practitioner wants to be notified when the results are available.

The nurse also documents if the test or procedure was performed and if the practitioner was notified according to the medical order. There are times when the test or procedure couldn't be performed as ordered, for example if the patient ate within 12 hours of the test when no food should have been eaten. In this situation, the nurse documents the reason for cancelling the test/procedure in this section and follows up with a further explanation in the nurse's notes.

	D	E	N
Tests/Procedures Results Reviewed by Physician			
Tests/Procedures CHEST X-RAY	AB		

Figure 4.7

4.4.2.5 Safety and Activity

This section (Figure 4.8) is used to specify the patient's permitted activity level based on the practitioner's orders. Activity levels are typically described as:

- Bed rest

- Bathroom privileges

- Out of bed ad lib

- Out of bed with assistance

- Physical therapy

	D	E	N
Activity Level: OOB	AB		
Safety: Call bell in reach	AB		
Number of Side Rails Up ____2__	AB		
Bed Position: Up Down	AB		
Call Bell Within Reach	AB		

Figure 4.8

Each shift, the nurse documents whether or not the patient complied with the activity level and if not, further explanation is provided in the nurse's notes.

Also specified in this section is whether or not the institution's safety protocol was adhered to. These typically include:

- Two side rails up

- Bed in the lowest position

- Call bell within reach

- Falls precaution

4.4.2.6 Discharge Plan

The Discharge Plan section (Figure 4.9) contains a very brief summary of where the patient is going after leaving the unit based on a needs assessment. It does not contain the complete patient's discharge plan, which is usually provided in a different document.

	D	E	N
Discharge Needs Assessment: Home _____1/1/08__ Rehab Facility _____ Subacute Facility _____	AB		
Transfer _____			
Discharge _____1/1/08_____	AB		

Figure 4.9

Items in the Discharge Plan section are:

- Home
- Rehabilitation facility
- Subacute facility
- Transfer
- Discharge

Solved Problems

4.1   What key information is contained in a care plan?

- The patient's problem(s)
- Interventions to address each problem
- The expected outcome or goal of these interventions
- Evaluation of the intervention

4.2   What is an action?

An action is taken by the healthcare team to minimize or resolve the patient's problems

4.3   What must be contained in an action?

- Must be based on a scientific rationale
- Have a measurable outcome
- Be patient specific

4.4   How is each patient problem described?

Each problem is described as a nursing diagnosis.

4.5   What is a nursing diagnosis?

A nursing diagnosis is a standardized statement defined by a recognized body such as the North American Nursing Diagnosis Association (NANDA).

4.6   What is the PES format?

The PES format has three components:

- **P** is the nursing diagnosis

- **E** is the etiology or origin of the problem

- **S** is the sign or symptoms that lead the healthcare team to choose this nursing diagnosis

4.7   What is a goal?

A goal is a measurable outcome that is expected after the healthcare team performs the action.

4.8   How is a goal assessed?

Each goal is assessed after the action is performed to determine if the desired result was achieved. The assessment is made using a standard measurement, which many times involves the patient reporting a condition or performing a behavior.

4.9   Give examples of a subjective and an objective measurement.

Measuring pain is subjective based on the patient's definition of pain. A temperature of 100°F is objective and is not influenced by interpretation.

4.10   How should an action be written?

Each action begins with a verb such as *assess, assist, explain*, and *teach* and is followed by the description of the action.

4.11   What is a scientific rationale?

It is the scientific basis for taking an action that is a recognized standard of practice and is documented in a healthcare facilities policy or by an authoritative source.

4.12   What is the evaluation?

Every action is evaluated to determine if the action impacted the patient and whether or not the goal was achieved.

4.13   How would you document if an outcome is not observed?

Write "not observed."

4.14   Are goals always 100 percent achieved?

Goals are not always 100 percent achieved. The level of achievement is indicated in the evaluation.

4.15   How is an outcome written?

The outcome is described in a sentence or paragraph that usually begins with *the patient* followed by an explanation of how the patient reacted to the action and if the goal associated with the action was reached.

4.16   What is a risk diagnosis?

Risk diagnosis consists of potential problems that the patient is at risk for developing and begins with *risk for*, such as *risk for injury*.

4.17   What is a possible diagnosis?

Possible diagnosis consists of problems that the patient may have, but there is insufficient information to make the diagnosis. This begins with *possible*, such as *possible fluid volume excess*.

4.18   What is a syndrome diagnosis?

Syndrome diagnosis is a problem that consists of a cluster of other diagnoses such as chronic pain.

4.19   What is a wellness diagnosis?

Wellness diagnosis consists of problems that could arise because of the patient's ill health and usually begins with *potential for*.

4.20   What are two common care plan formats?

Nursing care plan and interdisciplinary care plan are two common care plan formats.

4.21   What is a nursing care plan?

It is a comprehensive style required by nursing schools.

4.22   What is an interdisciplinary care plan?

An interdisciplinary care plan is a comprehensive, interdisciplinary plan that identifies care over a 24-hour period delivered by all members of the patient's healthcare team.

4.23   What is a care map?

This is another term for interdisciplinary care plan.

4.24   What are the categories of an interdisciplinary care plan?

- Nutrition

- Assessment and treatment

- Teaching and psychosocial

- Specimens and diagnostics

- Safety and activity

- Discharge plan

4.25   What is the purpose of the safety and activity section of the interdisciplinary care plan?

This section is used to specify the patient's permitted activity level based on the practitioner's orders.

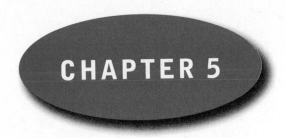

CHAPTER 5

The Words of Charting

5.1   Definition

A key responsibility of a nurse is to assess the patient for objective and subjective data and then translate the results of the assessment into terms that accurately describe the patient's condition. These terms are then written into the patient's chart so that other members of the patient's healthcare team can identify the patient's problems and devise a care plan for the patient.

Both printed and electronic charts contain lists of words used to describe common patient assessments. The nurse selects the appropriate words from the list that best describe the patient's assessment.

In addition both printed and electronic charts provide a blank form called a progress note where the nurse comes up with the proper words to describe the patient's assessment. Selecting the proper words to use is critical to conveying the nurse's assessment to members of the healthcare team.

5.2   Charting Your Assessment

Depending on the type of charting required by the healthcare institution, the healthcare provider will chart both normal and exceptional findings of the patient's assessment or chart only the exceptions. Many healthcare institutions use charting by exception because it reduces the time necessary to chart and the volume of information in the chart.

Abbreviations are frequently used when charting as a way to reduce the time and space needed to write your notes. Table 5.1 shows some abbreviations that are commonly used. Check the healthcare facility's list of approved and prohibited abbreviations as published by the Joint Commission with regard to the patient safety goals.

Healthcare facilities decide on the method to describe the patient's assessment in the chart. At times the nurse may be asked to tell how he or she found the patient when entering the room. The nurse might write:

Patient in bed, awake, alert and oriented times 3, bed in low position, 2 side rails up, call bell in reach, daughter at bedside. ID band on.

This description is then followed by a head-to-toe assessment of the patient as shown in Figure 5.1. The remaining pages of this chapter contain words and phrases that can be used to describe the patient's condition.

TABLE 5.1 Abbreviations Used in Charting

ABBREVIATION	DESCRIPTION	ABBREVIATION	DESCRIPTION
PT	Patient	R in a circle	Right
SR	Side rails	LW	Left wrist
RM	Room	RW	Right wrist
Bilat	Bilateral	BR	Bathroom
		BRP	Bathroom privilege
L in a circle	Left	BM	Bowel movement
OOB	Out of Bed	P	Pulse
Resp	Respiration	T	Temperature
BP	Blood pressure	Cap refill	Capillary refill
AC	Antecubital	S with a line over	Without
A&O	Alert and oriented	C with a line over	With
CTA	Clear to auscultation	WNL	Within normal limits

Progress Notes

19:00 PT in bed, low position. HOB 30 degrees. 2 SR↑. Call bell in reach. ID ban on. Bed rest. Wife at bedside. NPO. BP 161/90 T 98.3 Rep 26 P 80 bounding. POX 96 on rm air. pain 2 (0-10), oriented X3, cooperative, PERL, smile symmetric, no deviation of tongue, no productive cough, lungs R upper lung wheezing, R lower, L clear telemetry #29 NSR. IV sit .45 NS 100 ml/hr L wrist heparin lock, 20 gauge clear, dry via pump. Cap refill < 3 sec, Hand grip equal, bowel sounds X4 quad, void + BM unassisted in bed pan. Pitting edema R Leg 1+ L Leg 1+. Equal pressure bilat feet, Pedal Pulse strong bilat. Wound L Inferior calf laceration with sutures clean dry intact. VAC dressing CDI to -125 mm Hg draining serosangunous drainage.

Figure 5.1

5.2.1 Appearance

5.2.1.1 Normal

- Posture (erect/relaxed)
- Body movement (voluntary/deliberate/coordinated/smooth and even)
- Dress (appropriate for setting, season, age, gender, social group/clothing fits)
- Grooming and hygiene (hair is neat and clean/facial hair shaved or well groomed/nails clean)

5.2.1.2 Abnormal

- Posture (curled in bed/darting watchful eyes/restless pacing/sitting slumped/dragging feet/slow walking/sitting at edge of bed)

- Body movement (restless/fidgety/facial grimace/unsteady gait/uncoordinated)

- Dress (inappropriate for setting, season, age, gender, social group/clothing does not fit)

- Grooming and hygiene (unilateral neglect/poor hygiene/lack of concern about dress/not groomed/disheveled)

5.2.2 Behavior

5.2.2.1 Normal

- Level of consciousness (awake/alert/aware/oriented/recent memory/judgment/mood/affect)

- Facial expression (appropriate/changes with topic/eye contact)

- Speech (effortlessly/clear/shares conversation/fluent/understandable/forms words/completes sentences/native language/articulation/pattern)

- Mood and affect (appropriate/cooperative)

5.2.2.2 Abnormal

- Level of consciousness (lethargic/obtunded/stupor/semicomatose/comatose/confused/disoriented)

- Facial expression (flat/masklike/grimacing)

- Mood and affect (flat)

- Speech (dysphonia/monopolizes conversation/silent/secretive/uncommunicative/slow/monotonus/rapid-fire/pressures/loud/dysarthria/misuses words/omits words/transposes words/repetitious/long delays in finding word/failure in word search/nonverbal/garbled)

- Mood and affect (flat/blunted/anxious/fearful/irritabile/rage/ambivalent/labile/euphoric/elation/depersonalization/depressed/dulled concentration/impaired judgment/uninhibited/talkative/impaired memory)

- Pain (as per pain scale)

5.2.3 Nutrition

5.2.3.1 Normal

- Skin (smooth/no rashes/no bruises/flaking/warm/dry)

- Hair (shiny/firm/healthy scalp)

- Eyes (clear/shiny/membranes pink and moist/no sores at corners of eyelids)

- Lips (smooth/not chapped/not swollen/pink/not cracked)

- Tongue (red/not swollen/not smooth/no lesions)

- Gums (reddish pink/firm/no swelling/no bleeding)
- Nails (smooth/pink/clean)

5.2.3.2 Abnormal

- Skin (dry/flaking/scaly/petechial/ecchymostic/bumpy/cracks/lesions/hyperpigmentation/rash/bruised/diaphoretic/cool/clammy)
- Hair (dull/dry/sparse/corkscrew hair/color changes/falls out easily)
- Eyes (dryness/pale conjunctivae/red conjunctivae/softening/foamy plaques)
- Lips (vertical cracks on lips/red cracks at sides of mouth)
- Tongue (beefy red/pale/papillary atrophy/papillary hypertrophy/purplish)
- Gums (bleeding)
- Nails (brittle/ridged/spoon-shaped/splintered/hemorrhages/striata/jagged/bitten/dirty/clubbing/cyanotic/spongy/pitted/transverse grooves/lines)

5.2.4 Vital Signs

5.2.4.1 Normal

- Pulse (write value)
- Blood pressure (write value)
- Pain (absent)

5.2.4.2 Abnormal

- Pulse (full/bounding/weak/thready/absent)
- Blood pressure (write abnormal value)
- Pain (burning/stabbing/aching/throbbing/firelike/squeezing/cramping/sharp/itching/tingling/shooting/crushing/dull/crying/moaning/pain when palpated/clutching area)

5.2.5 Skin

5.2.5.1 Normal

- Color (freckle [ephelis]/mole [nevus]/junctional nevus/birthmark/diameter in millimeters/senile lentigines)
- IV sites (clean, dry, intact with no signs of redness/no signs of infiltration)
- Temperature (write temperature)

- Moisture (warm/dry)

- Texture (smooth/soft/no dryness/no cracking/no rashes)

- Thickness (normal/uniform)

- Edema (none)

- Turgor (no tenting)

5.2.5.2 Abnormal

- Color (brown/tan/black-blue [ecchymosis]/red (erythema)/white/yellow/ashen gray/asymmetrical pigment/border notching/border scalloping/border ragged edges/border poorly defined margins/pencil eraser–size/elevated/keratosis)

- Dressings (wound drainage: serosanguineous, purulent, sanguineous, scant/saturated/red-brown)

- IV sites (not clean, not dry, not intact/signs of redness/infiltration, cool, swollen/phlebitis, red, warm to touch)

- Temperature (hyperthermia/hypothermia)

- Moisture (diaphoresis/dry/parched/cracked)

- Texture (velvetlike/rough/dry/flaky/blisters)

- Thickness (very thin/shiny/atrophic/callus)

- Edema (1+/2+/3+/4+ pitting)

- Turgor (tenting)

5.2.6 Lesions

5.2.6.1 Normal

- Description (no lesions)

5.2.6.2 Abnormal

- Description (annular/circular/begins in center/spreads/runs together/confluent/discrete/distinct/ grouped/clustered/target/polycyclic/together/zosteriform/linear arrangement/linear/scratch/streak/line/ stripe/gyrate/twisted/coiled/spiral/snakelike/flat/less than/greater than/solid/elevated/hard/soft/deep/ shallow/superficial/raised/transient/dried-out exudate/honey-colored/weeping/shedding/silver/ micalike/yellow/greasy/depressed/smooth/rubbery/clawlike)

- Type (macule/patch/nodule/wheal/fluid held/urticaria/hives/vesicle/bulla/cyst/pustule/crust/scale/ linear crack/abrupt edges/fissure/erosion/ulcer/scar/lichenification/prolonged intense scratching/ excoriation/atrophic scar/keloid/hypertrophic scar/port-wine stain/strawberry mark/spider/star/ purpura/petechiae/venous lake)

5.2.7 Eyes

5.2.7.1 Normal

- Eyes (iris intact/conjunctivae clear/sclerae white/cornea intact/ PERRLA [pupils equal round reactive to light and accommodation])

5.2.7.2 Abnormal

- Eyes (lower lid dropping away/lower lid turning in/lids edematous/discolored/swollen/almost shut/inward turn of eye/outward turn of eye/inward drift/outward drift/periorbital edema/protruding eyes/drooping upper lid/light-colored areas in outer iris/large space between eyes/inflammation of eyelids/stye/inflammation of lacrimal sac/nodule protruding on lid/infective conjunctivae/ circumcorneal redness/subconjunctival hemorrhage/corneal abrasion/unequal pupil/constricted pupils/fixed pupils/sluggish reaction to light/enlarged pupils/pupils no response to light)

5.2.8 Ears

5.2.8.1 Normal

- Ears (no tenderness/no discharge/no masses/no lesions/canals clear of cerumen/able to hear whispered voice bilaterally)

5.2.8.2 Abnormal

- Ears (reddish blue discoloration of auricle/swelling/skin tag/painful movement of the pinna/purulent discharge/scaling/itching/clear fluid discharge/infected hair follicle)

5.2.9 Nose, Mouth, Throat

5.2.9.1 Normal

- Nose (naris patent/mucosa pink/nontender/no lesions/no obstruction/mobile/no discharge/no swelling)
- Mouth and throat (mucosa pink/no lesions/uvula midline/rises on phonation/tonsils present/no lumps on tonsils)

5.2.9.2 Abnormal

- Nose (mucosa gray and boggy/tender/lesions/obstruction/not mobile/discharge)
- Mouth and throat (coated tongue/dry mouth/absent salivation/decreased salivation/increased salivation/lesions/plaque/pain/ulcers/vesicles/purulent drainage/hemorrhagic/edema/no tonsils/ coughing/aspiration/regurgitation/white, cheesy curdlike patch/chalky-white, thick raised patches/borders well defined/blue-white spots/irregular red halo)

5.2.10   Breasts

5.2.10.1   Normal

- Location (upper inner quadrant/upper outer quadrant/lower inner quadrant/lower outer quadrant/auxiliary tail of Spence)

5.2.10.2   Abnormal

- Breasts (thickening/swelling/changes in bra size/rash/tenderness/hyperpigmentation/dimpling/pucker)
- Discharge (color/thick/runny/odor/first noticed)
- Lump (location/width/length/thickness/oval/round/lobulated/indistinct/soft/firm/hard/movable/fixed/single/multiple/erythematous/dimpled/retracted/tender)

5.2.11   Lungs

5.2.11.1   Normal

- Location (anterior axillary line/midclavicular line/midsternal line/scapular line/vertebral line/posterior axillary line/midaxillary line/right upper lobe [RUL]/right middle lobe [RML])/right lower lobe [RLL]/left upper lobe [LUL]/left lower lobe [LLL])
- Palpation (chest symmetrical/tactile fremitus equal bilaterally/no lumps/no tenderness)
- Resonance (equal bilaterally)
- Adventitious sounds (none/clear to auscultation/clear to all lung fields)
- Respirations even, non-labored

5.2.11.2   Abnormal

- Cough (continuous/afternoon/evenings/night/early morning/streaks of blood/frank blood/sputum production/color/amount/hacking/dry/barking/hoarse/congested/bubbling/occurs on lying)
- Respiration (shortness of breath/hard breathing/shallow/tachypnea/bradypnea/hyperventilation/hypoventilation/Cheyne-Stokes)
- Tactile fremitus (decrease/increase/rhonchal/pleural friction/crepitus/crackling)
- Resonance (dull/hyperresonance)
- Adventitious sounds (fine crackles/coarse crackles/rales/pleural friction rub/wheeze on inspiration or expiration or both/stridor/rhonchi/absent or decreased or diminished)

5.2.12 Cardiac

5.2.12.1 Normal

- Chest pain (none)
- Skin (pink)
- Carotid artery (no bruit/normal pulse/no distention)
- Pain (no pain)

5.2.12.2 Abnormal

- Chest pain (crushing/stabbing/burning/viselike/duration)
- Causes of pain (rest/emotional upset/after eating/during intercourse/cold weather)
- Pain increases (moving arm/moving neck/breathing/lying flat)
- Associated symptoms (pale skin/skips beat/shortness of breath/nausea/vomiting/fast rate/number of pillows used to sleep)
- Skin (ashen/pallor/cyanosis/cool, clammy/diaphoretic)
- Carotid artery (bruit/diminished pulse/increased pulse/strong pulse/distention/bounding)

5.2.13 Peripheral Vascular

5.2.13.1 Normal

- Skin (pink)
- Visualized veins (none observed)
- Cramp (none)

5.2.13.2 Abnormal

- Cramp (burning/aching/stabbing/gradual/sudden/awakens at night/worse in cool weather/worse when elevated)
- Cramp relieved by (dangling/walking/rubbing/stopping walking)
- Skin (red/pallor/blue/brown)
- Visualized veins (bulging/crooked/ulcerated/swollen/distended/torturous)

5.2.14 Gastrointestinal

5.2.14.1 Normal

- Food intolerance (none)
- Stomach/abdominal pain (none)
- Bowel (last BM/well formed/normal color/bowel sounds present x 4)
- Appetite (normal)
- Weight (no change)
- Abdominal contour (flat/rounded/obese)
- Abdomen (no mass/no tenderness/soft/not tender/not distended)

5.2.14.2 Abnormal

- Food intolerance (heartburn/belching/bloating/indigestion/allergic reaction)
- Stomach/abdominal pain (moves around/aggravated by movement/dull/general/poorly localized/sharp/precisely localized/aggravating factors/alleviating factors/difficulty swallowing/bulging location/firm/rigid/distended/guarded)
- Bowel (last BM/tarry stool/red stool/gray stool)
- Appetite (loss of appetite)
- Weight (unexpected increase/unexpected decrease)
- Abdominal contour (scalphoid/protuberant)
- Abdomen (dull/distended/hyperresonance/pulsating/systolic bruit)

5.2.15 Musculoskeletal

5.2.15.1 Normal

- Joint (no tenderness/no swelling/full ROM/no stiffness/no deformity/not tender)

5.2.15.2 Abnormal

- Joint (redness/swelling/heat/tenderness/limited ROM/stiffness/tender/nodules/deformity)

5.2.16 Neurologic

5.2.16.1 Normal (see also Behavior)

- Head/mental status (alert/oriented to person, place, time/cooperative/recent memory/judgment/mood/affect/speech clarity/articulation/pattern/content appropriate/native language/facial expression/PERRLA [pupils equal, round, reactive to light. and accommodation])

- Peripherals (dorsiflexion/plantar flexion/reflex)
- Gait (tandem walking/smooth/rhythmic/effortless/coordinated)

5.2.16.2 Abnormal

- Head (headache/dizziness/lightheaded/vertigo/patient's feeling of spinning/feeling that room is spinning/syncope/aura/seizures/shaking/difficulty speaking/difficulty swallowing/uncoordinated/lethargic/obtunded/stupor/semicomatose/delirium)
- Peripherals (tremors/burning/tingling/numbness/muscle weakness)
- Gait (stiff/unsteady/rigid arms/ataxia/staggering/crooked line of walk)

Solved Problems

5.1   Why is it important to use the proper wording in a patient's chart?

Selecting the proper word to use is critical to conveying the nurse's assessment to members of the healthcare team.

5.2   What type of chart would require a nurse to select the wording of the assessment?

A progress note because progress notes are free formed text.

5.3   What kind of charting is commonly used in healthcare institutions?

Charting by exception is commonly used in healthcare institutions.

5.4   What is charting by exception?

Only abnormal findings in a patient's assessment are charted.

5.5   What is the advantage of charting by exception?

It reduces the time and space necessary to write a patient's assessment.

5.6   Can abbreviations be used in charting?

Yes, if the healthcare facility approves and the abbreviations are approved by the Joint Commission with regard to the patient safety goals.

5.7   What is another kind of charting that is used in nursing schools and has limited use by healthcare facilities?

This would be head-to-toe patient assessment.

5.8   What is head-to-toe patient assessment charting?

The nurse charts the patient's assessment of both normal and abnormal findings.

5.9   What are the common assessments made of a patient's appearance?

Posture, body movement, dress, grooming, and hygiene are the common assessments made of a patient's appearance.

5.10   What words might be used to describe a patient's abnormal body movement?

Restless/fidgety/facial grimace/unsteady gait/uncoordinated.

5.11   What words might be used to describe a patient's abnormal posture?

Curled in bed/darting watchful eyes/restless pacing/sitting slumped/dragging feet/slow walking/sitting at edge of bed.

5.12   What are the common assessments made of a patient's behavior?

Level of consciousness, facial expression, speech, mood and affect.

5.13   What words might be used to describe a patient's abnormal level of consciousness?

Lethargic/obtunded/stupor/semicoma/coma/confused/disoriented.

5.14   What words might be used to describe a patient's abnormal speech?

Dysphonia/monopolizes conversation/silent/secretive/uncommunicative/slow/monotonus/rapid-fire/pressures/loud/dysarthria/misuses words/omits words/transposes words/repetitious/long delays in finding words/failure in word search/nonverbal/garbled.

5.15   What words might be used to describe a patient's abnormal mood and affect?

Flat/blunted/anxious/fearful/irritable/enraged/ambivalent/ labile/euphoric/elated/depersonalized/depressed/dulled concentration/impaired judgment/uninhibited/talkativeness/impaired memory.

5.16   What are the common assessments made of a patient's nutrition?

Skin, hair, eyes, lips, tongue, gums, and nails.

5.17   What words might be used to describe a patient's abnormal skin?

Dry/flaking/scaly/petechiae/ecchymoses/bumpy/cracks/lesion/hyperpigmentation/rash/bruise.

5.18   What words might be used to describe a patient's abnormal tongue?

Beefy red/pale/papillary atrophy/papillary hypertrophy/purplish.

5.19   What words might be used to describe a patient's abnormal hair?

Dull/dry/sparse/corkscrew hair/color changes/falls out easily.

5.20 What words might be used to describe a patient's pain?

Burning/stabbing/aching/throbbing/firelike/squeezing/cramping/sharp/itching/tingling/shooting/
crushing/dull/crying/moaning/pain when palpated/clutching area.

5.21 What words might be used to describe a patient's abnormal IV site?

Not clean, not dry, not intact/signs of redness/infiltration, cool, swollen/phlebitis, red, warm to touch.

5.22 What words might be used to describe a patient's abnormal lesion?

Annular/circular/begins in center/spreads/runs together/confluent/discrete/distinct/grouped/clustered/
target/polycyclic/together/zosteriform/linear arrangement/linear/scratch/streaked/lined/striped/gyrated/
twisted/coiled/spiralled/snakelike/flat/less than/greater than/solid/elevated/hard/soft/deep/shallow/
superficial/raised/transient/dried-out exudate/honey-colored/weeping/shedding/silver/micalike/
yellow/greasy/depressed/smooth/rubbery/clawlike.

5.23 What words might be used to describe a patient's abnormal lesion type?

Macule/patch/nodule/wheal/fluid held/urticaria/hives/vesicle/bulla/cyst/pustule/crust/scale/linear
crack/abrupt edges/fissure/erosion/ulcer/scar/lichenification/prolonged intense scratching/excoriation/
atrophic scar/keloid/hypertrophic scar/port-wine stain/strawberry mark/spider/star/purpura/petechiae/
venous lake.

5.24 What words might be used to describe a patient's abnormal eyes?

Lower lid dropping away/lower lid turning in/lids edematous/discolored/swollen/almost shut/inward
turn of eye/outward turn of eye/inward drift/outward drift/periorbital edema/protruding eyes/drooping
upper lid/light-colored areas in outer iris/large space between eyes/inflammation of eyelids/stye
/inflammation of lacrimal sac/nodule protruding on lid/infective conjunctivae/circumcorneal redness/
subconjunctival hemorrhage/corneal abrasion/unequal pupil/constricted pupils/fixed pupils/sluggish
reaction to light/enlarged pupils/pupils no response to light.

5.25 What words might be used to describe a patient's abnormal mouth and throat?

Coated tongue/dry mouth/absent salivation/decreased salivation/increased salivation/lesions/plaque/
pain/ulcers/vesicles/purulent drainage/hemorrhagic/edema/no tonsils/coughing/aspiration/
regurgitation/white, cheesy curdlike patch/chalky-white, thick raised patches/borders well
defined/blue-white spots/irregular red halo.

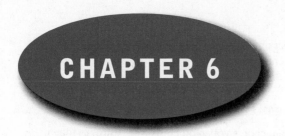

CHAPTER 6

Computer Charting

6.1 Definition

Computer charts provide an efficient way to record and share patient information. Computer charts are still vulnerable to many of the same errors as paper charts and can introduce new errors into a patient's record.

There are three tasks necessary for computer charting:

- Know which keys to press

- Know what happens to patient information after those keys are pressed

- Practice charting patient information

6.2 Computer Charting System Components

The computer screen is just one of many parts of a computer charting system. The other parts are hidden from sight because they are not needed to use the computer charting system.

There are six major parts of a computer charting system. These are:

- Computer workstation

- Network

- Server

- Database

- Printers

- Charting program

6.2.1 Computer Workstation

A computer workstation is a PC (personal computer) used to chart patient information. Some healthcare facilities have a PC at each nurse's station and others also have a laptop PC that can be moved to the patient's room. Although they are referred to as a computer workstation in the healthcare facility, these are the same PCs that might be found at home.

A PC, or any computer for that matter, is a box of switches (see Workstation: An Inside Look). A special group of computer programs called an operating system enables those switches to store and manipulate information. Arguably the most widely used operating system is Microsoft Windows, found on many home computers. This operating system is used on most workstations in healthcare facilities.

6.2.2 Network

Workstations are connected together by a computer network (see Network: An Inside Look) called an intranet (Figure 6.1). Think of a network as a highway over which patient information travels. The network is a highway of cables that stretch from each workstation through the walls and floors and into a central room called a data center that contains other computers called servers (see Server) that consolidate patient information into a database (see Database).

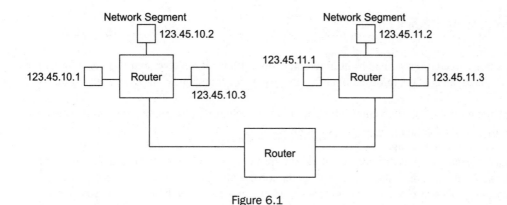

Figure 6.1

Some workstations might be connected to the network through a wireless connection called Wi-Fi, where patient information is transmitted to a receiver that is connected to the network via a cable. This is the same way a favorite song is transmitted by a radio station to an individual radio. The only difference is that the Wi-Fi transmitter sends encrypted (see Encryption) patient information within the healthcare facility.

6.2.3 Database

A database is a collection of data. A patient's database is created by gathering objective and subjective information about the patient through assessment. With computerized charting, the database is an electronic collection of data from all patients.

Think of the database as an electronic filing cabinet containing patient information that can be stored and accessed using a workstation over the healthcare facility's computer network. This is very similar to how a person can access his bank account information from his home PC over the Internet.

6.2.4   Printers

The trend is to replace printing information on paper with displaying the information on a computer screen. However, realistically some print is still necessary, which is why a printer can also be found at the nurses' station.

A printer is connected to the network enabling workstations to share the same printer. In addition, workstations can use other printers on the network by choosing a printer from a list of available printers (see Chapter 7). If the printer at a particular nurses' station isn't working, the printer at the nearest nurses' station can be used.

6.2.5   Charting Program

The term *computer program* is familiar to anyone who has used a home computer. There are many computer programs available, each of which allows the computer to do something unique, such as word processing using Microsoft Word.

A charting program allows the computer to record, retrieve, edit, and print a patient's chart. There are many different kinds of charting programs available, all of which are used to electronically chart patient information; however each does so in a slightly different way. In the next chapter the features found in many charting programs will be explained.

6.3   Workstation: An Inside Look

A workstation is similar to a computer and is used to enter, store, transmit, receive, and display information such as emails, web pages, and patient information. It has many features found on a computer, enabling easy use of the workstation.

The keyboard and mouse are used to enter information into the charting program and other programs that the healthcare facility has on the workstation. However, there are also other devices used to input data, such as a bar code reader that is used in the supermarket.

A bar code reader scans bar codes that contain encoded information that is translated into data that is understandable. Depending on the nature of the charting program, a bar code reader is used to scan employee IDs, patient ID bracelets, bar codes on medication, laboratory specimens, and medical supplies. This saves time entering information into the workstation and increases the accuracy of the information by reducing the risk of typographical errors.

For example, before administering medication, the nurse scans her employee ID, scans the medication, and scans the patient's ID bracelet into the workstation. The workstation then verifies that the correct medication and dose is going to be administered to the right patient at the right time using the prescribed method of administration. A warning message is displayed if there is a discrepancy. If all the information is correct, the nurse then uses the keyboard or mouse to confirm that the medication was administered.

6.3.1   Where the Information Goes

The information is temporarily stored in the workstation's memory and is sometimes also stored on the workstation's hard drive. Information stored in memory is erased automatically when the workstation is turned off. Information stored on the hard drive remains on the hard drive even after the workstation is turned off.

Many charting programs automatically transmit information over the network to a data center rather than storing information on the workstation's hard drive, eliminating the worry of losing information. This is done for security reasons.

Furthermore, workstations are typically powered by circuits that are connected to the healthcare facility's backup power supplies. Workstations remain operating during a power outage.

6.3.2 Retrieving and Displaying Information

In order to recall and display information, the healthcare provider will be prompted to enter his or her ID and password that are provided by the healthcare facility. This ID is granted rights to retrieve and display information the healthcare provider is authorized to view based on HIPAA (Health Insurance Portability and Accountability Act) and the healthcare facility's policy. The healthcare facility's technology department assigns those rights.

For example, after the nurse enters his or her ID and password (logging in), the charting program displays a list of patients assigned by the nurse manager. The nurse is able to access information about those patients needed to do his or her job. The charting program automatically hides unauthorized information.

Access to patient information might be limited. It is common for the workstation to automatically erase information from the screen and log out the healthcare provider after a period of time has passed to assure that the information remains secure. This reduces the risk that patient information can be viewed on the screen after the nurse walks away from the workstation or that another person can use the workstation while the nurse is still logged in.

6.3.3 Demystifying Data

If the nurse is curious as to how words are stored inside the workstation, then reading this section will be helpful; otherwise it can be skipped.

The workstation contains tiny electronic switches that can be turned on or off—similar to a light switch. In order to store a character found on the keyboard to the workstation, the character must first be translated into a number that consists of a series of 0s and 1s called a binary number. This probably sounds too nerdy, but it is easy to understand.

There is a code book that assigns each keyboard character a binary number. When a key on the keyboard is pressed, a program inside the workstation looks up the letter in the code book and then reads the corresponding binary number.

Let's see how this works. Enter the word *nurse* into the workstation and these letters are translated in the binary numbers shown in Table 6.1.

TABLE 6.1

ACSII BINARY	ALPHABET
110 1110	n
111 0101	u
111 0010	r
111 0011	s
110 0101	e

The next step is storing these binary numbers into the electronic switches inside the workstation. Imagine for a moment that each switch is a light switch that can be turned off and on. Let's say the off position is zero and the on position is one. Several light switches can be grouped together and its setting can be used to store a keyboard character.

Take a look at the first letter in Table 6.1. Each digit represents a light switch. The first two light switches are on, the third is off, the next three are on, and the last is off. By setting these switches accordingly, the letter "n" is stored inside the workstation.

The workstation displays keyboard characters by translating the switch settings (binary numbers) into images on the screen. The workstation screen is made up of tiny dots called pixels (picture elements). Think of these as tiny lightbulbs. There are millions of them on a screen.

A program inside the workstation reads the setting of the light switches and then turns on the appropriate lightbulbs on the screen to create the image of the corresponding keyboard character.

6.4   Network: An Inside Look

A computer network is a highway that connects together workstations, printers, and computing devices in the healthcare facility's data center. The network can also extend to physician offices, paramedic mobile units, Medevac aircraft, and organizations that do business with the healthcare facility, such as insurance companies, banks, and suppliers.

Any computing device (i.e., workstation) on the network can transmit data to another computing device by sending data over the network. For example, a practitioner can use the workstation at the nurse's station to send a medication order over the network to the pharmacy.

6.4.1   The Network Is a Hometown

How does this electronic highway work? It works like a hometown. Each workstation, printer, and other computing devices has a unique address called an IP address. Think of this as the address of a house. The street is the pathway to buildings in the town, similar to how the network cable is the pathway to computing devices on the network.

When a friend wants to send another friend who lives across town an invitation to a barbeque, he places the invitation in an envelope and writes on the envelope the friend's address as the destination address and his own address as the return address, and then gives the envelope to the postal carrier who is driving down the street. The postal carrier delivers the envelope to that town's post office where the envelope is sorted and given to the friend's postal carrier who delivers it to the friend's house.

This is basically the same process that occurs when data are sent over a computer network. The envelope is an electronic envelope called a packet. The data that are to be sent are electronically placed into the packet, and the packet is addressed with the destination computer's IP address and the IP address of the computer sending the packet. The packet is then sent along the network to a post office–like device called a router where the packet is then forwarded to the destination computer.

A computer network typically has several "towns," each referred to as a network segment (see Figure 6.1). Segments are connected to regional routers (regional post offices) via cable enabling data to be easily transmitted to any network segment.

This is similar to how a county or parish is divided into many towns. Towns are connected together by county roads. And mail sent to a different town is first sent from the town's post office to a regional post office, where it is redirected to the other town's post office, which delivers the letter to its destination address.

6.4.2   How Words Move Along a Cable

If the healthcare provider is curious as to how the electronic envelope travels across the network cable, be sure to read this section; otherwise it can be skipped.

Imagine for a moment a dishpan filled with water. The water is still. A wave can be created in the dishpan by moving a knife up and down in the water. Each time the knife is pushed down, water molecules are moved up, creating the wave. No wave is created when the knife is out of the water.

The 0s and 1s used to represent characters on the keyboard (see Demystifying Data) can be represented by a wave. The peak of the wave is 1, and no wave is 0 (Figure 6.2). By pushing—and withholding—the knife in the water a keyboard character can be transmitted across the dishpan.

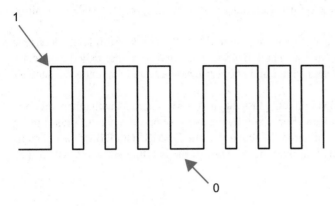

Figure 6.2

Although this isn't very practical, it illustrates the concept used to transmit 0s and 1s over network cables. In networks, an electronic wave is created when electricity is applied to the cable. The electricity is controlled by circuits inside the computer that translates the 0s and 1s of the electronic envelope into the wave. Circuits in the destination computer translate electronic waves back to 0s and 1s and store them in switches inside the computer.

6.4.2.1 Transmitting Without Cable

A customer using a laptop to surf the net at a table in an upscale coffee shop doesn't need a cable to connect to the Internet because the coffee shop provided a Wi-Fi connection—a wireless connection to the Internet.

Healthcare facilities are also using Wi-Fi technology to connect laptops to the healthcare facility's network. Laptops are mobile workstations that can be brought to each patient's room, enabling the nurse to update the patient's chart immediately after caring for the patient.

Wi-Fi uses radio waves, which is the same technology used to broadcast radio programs only over a very short distance. Laptops and other mobile computing devices have a built-in Wi-Fi transceiver. This consists of circuits that can transmit a signal and receive a signal. Any receiver tuned to the Wi-Fi's frequency can receive the signal, but only authorized receivers can understand the data that are being transmitted.

All data are encrypted before being transmitted. Only a receiver with the proper cipher can decipher the data, and in this way protects the data from eavesdropping computer devices that connect to Wi-Fi.

6.4.3 Demystifying Wi-Fi Transmission

This section is for the nurse who is inquisitive about how data are transmitted through the air using Wi-Fi transmission.

Remember back to third grade science class when the teacher said there are molecules of air all around even though they cannot be seen or felt. Air molecules are similar to water molecules that were moved with the knife in the earlier example to create a wave in the dishpan (see How Words Move Along a Cable). Air molecules are pushed to create a wave.

Circuits in the Wi-Fi transceiver, located inside a computing device, set air molecules in motion, creating a wave. 0s and 1s are encoded by designating the peak of a wave as 1 and no wave or the bottom of the wave as 0.

Wi-Fi technology replaces the cable in a network. Other network features such as the electronic envelope (packet) and IP addresses are used. The electronic envelope is transmitted over the Wi-Fi signal.

6.5   Database: An Inside Look

The patient's chart, patient billing, payroll, and employee information are just a few types of information that a healthcare facility must store and retrieve quickly in order to care for patients and pay their own bills. Most information is stored electronically, although some information must be stored in its original state as required by the healthcare facility's legal department.

Electronic information is stored in a database management system (DBMS). Think of this as an electronic filing cabinet and a super–file clerk all rolled up in one. The DBMS resides on a computer called a database server that is located in the healthcare facility's data center and is operated by a technician called a database administrator.

It is rare that a healthcare provider uses a DBMS directly. Instead, the DBMS interacts with other software, such as the charting software used to care for patients. For example, the nurse selects the patient's chart using the charting software and the charting software forwards the request to the DBMS. The DBMS searches its records for the information and sends the information over the network to the charting software, which then displays the information on the screen.

6.5.1   Security Access

HIPAA and other regulations, in addition to good business practices, require that access to a healthcare facility's computers and information stored in those computers be restricted on a need-to-know basis. Restrictions are enforced by setting security access for each employee to the healthcare facility's computers.

Each employee who is permitted access to the healthcare facility's computers is assigned a unique user ID and password. Behind the scenes, the user ID is permitted to access computer programs and information that corresponds to the security access settings assigned by the healthcare facility's information technology (IT) department.

6.5.1.1   User ID and Passwords

The IT department assigns the user IDs and creates temporary passwords. The healthcare provider is prompted to change the password the first time he or she logs into the computer. Only the healthcare provider knows the password. The IT department cannot access the new password.

The nurse enters her user ID and password into the computer in order to use the charting program. These are validated by the computer against a known user ID and password.

A rejection message is displayed if there is a mismatch of user ID and password or if the user ID is inaccurate. Often there is another opportunity to enter the correct user ID and password, depending on the healthcare facility's security access policy. At some point, the user ID will become suspended if it continues to be rejected. Typically, this occurs after three failed attempts.

The IT department can reinstate a user ID and password once it is satisfied the healthcare provider's identity has been properly verified. The healthcare facility's policy dictates how this is done. For example, the healthcare provider might have to visit the IT department and show an employee ID card. The ID department then resets the password to a temporary password. The worker will have to change the password the next time he or she logs into the computer.

6.5.2   Log in Frequently

There is a tendency to log into the computer, enter some information into the charting program, and then walk away from the computer to perform other patient care. This is a security risk for the healthcare facility because anyone could step up and use the computer without having to log in.

To prevent this unauthorized access, the IT department usually logs out a user ID automatically after a specific time period of idleness has transpired, such as every 10 minutes. The user ID isn't suspended. It can be used again to log back into the computer.

6.5.3 Encryption

Encryption is a process of converting information to a meaningless series of letters and numbers that can be stored or transmitted with little chance of anyone who doesn't have the cipher being able to convert it back to readable information.

At the heart of the conversion process is a mathematical formula that uses a value called a key to transform meaningful information into meaningless information (encryption) and meaningless information to meaningful information (decipher).

Healthcare information is encrypted using a 128-bit key. The more bits in a key, the harder it is to break the encryption. A bit is a 0 or 1 (see Demystifying Data). It isn't necessary to know any more about encryption because this is handled behind the scenes.

6.5.4 Hide Information in Plain Sight

Protecting patient information is challenging when the information is stored and accessed electronically. A major concern occurs when the information is displayed on the computer screen. Anyone walking in sight of the computer screen can view patient information displayed on the screen.

Healthcare facilities reduce the likelihood that the screen can be inappropriately viewed by automatically displaying a screen saver after a specified amount of time has passed. A screen saver is an image that is displayed when the computer is idle for a period of time. The healthcare facility's policy dictates the time period.

Another common technique used by healthcare facilities is to use a privacy filter over the screen. A privacy filter prevents anyone except the person in front of the computer from clearly seeing the image on the screen.

6.5.5 Limiting Control

Healthcare organizations whose stocks are traded publicly must comply with the Sarbanes Oxley (SOX) Act. SOX was enacted in response to corporate scandals such as with Enron. SOX basically requires that checks and balance control must be implemented and enforced using computers. These are sometimes referred to as SOX controls. SOX controls are mostly used for a publicly traded company.

A SOX control means that two or more persons should be responsible to complete a process to assure that one person does not have the capability to control a process from beginning to end. For example, a registered nurse (RN) can't reassign herself to another patient. This reassignment must be performed by the nurse manager.

6.5.6 Protecting Electronic Information

Patient information and other information needed for the healthcare facility to operate (i.e., billing information) are stored in databases in the healthcare facility's data center. The data center is especially designed to withstand many disasters such as power outages and fire.

Copies of databases and software such as the charting software are also stored off the premises in highly protected facilities usually operated by a vendor. These copies can be retrieved within hours should the on-site database become inaccessible.

In addition, some healthcare facilities have a duplicate contingency data center off premises that is immediately activated should the primary data center become unavailable.

6.6 A Tour of the IT Department

The healthcare provider will probably have some encounter with the healthcare facility's IT department whether it is to have an ID or password reset or to serve on an advisory committee to help select a charting program.

Therefore, it is probably a good idea to know how the IT department operates. The size and complexity of the IT department depends on the size of the healthcare facility. Larger facilities typically have more elaborate IT departments.

There are five groups found in most healthcare facility's IT departments. These are end user services, network, databases, applications, and administration.

The end user services group is responsible for the computer equipment on the unit and in the offices. This group is called whenever anything goes wrong with the workstation or if new equipment needs to be ordered.

The network group is responsible for the hardware and software that is necessary to send and receive information over the computer network. Typically, they are called by the end user services group whenever there is a problem with the network. That is, the healthcare provider will call the end user services group when his workstation isn't working properly. They in turn call the network group if the trouble is with the network and not the workstation.

The database group is in charge of maintaining electronic information. It is their job to make sure that the patient's information is securely stored and is available to the patient's healthcare team at a keystroke.

The applications group is in control of specialty programs such as the charting program that runs on all computers in the healthcare facility. They are the in-house experts who are called for assistance using that program.

The administration group sets the IT strategies and policies for the healthcare facility and oversees the operation of the other four groups within the IT division.

6.6.1   Outside Help

Healthcare facilities frequently employ the services of outside IT experts to supplement their in-house staff. These are referred to as outsourced services because they involve IT tasks that are handled by a vendor rather than by the healthcare facility's employees.

Some healthcare facilities find outsourcing an economical way to provide IT services. For example, it might be less expensive to call in a repair technician to fix a workstation than to have the technician on staff because workstations don't frequently malfunction.

The degree to which IT services are outsourced greatly depends on the size of the healthcare facility. Small healthcare facilities are unable to afford a broad-skilled IT staff and therefore find it financially sound to outsource most of the IT services. In contrast, larger healthcare facilities have a greater demand for these services and find it economical to have an in-house staff.

Solved Problems

6.1   What are the major parts of a computer charting system?

- Computer workstation

- Network

- Server

- Database

- Printers

- Charting program

6.2   What is a computer workstation?

A computer workstation is a PC (personal computer) used to chart patient information.

6.3   What is a network?

Workstations are connected together by a computer network. A network is like a highway over which patient information travels.

6.4   What is a wireless connection?

Some workstations might be connected to the network through a wireless connection called Wi-Fi, where patient information is transmitted to a receiver that is connected to the network via a cable.

6.5   What is a database?

A database is a collection of data. The database is like an electronic filing cabinet containing patient information that can be stored and accessed using a workstation over the healthcare facility's computer network.

6.6   What is a charting program?

A charting program allows the healthcare provider to use the computer to record, retrieve, edit, and print a patient's chart.

6.7   What is a bar code reader?

A bar code reader scans bar codes that contain encoded information and are translated into data that is understandable.

6.8   What rights to patient information are assigned to a healthcare provider's user ID?

The ID is granted rights to retrieve and display information that the healthcare provider is authorized to view based on HIPAA (Health Insurance Portability and Accountability Act) and the healthcare facility's policy.

6.9   What is an IP address?

An IP address is an address on the network assigned to a device that is connected to the network.

6.10   What is a packet?

A packet is an electronic envelope that is transmitted over a network.

6.11   What is a network segment?

A network segment is a smaller network within the network similar to towns within a state.

6.12   What is a router?

A router connects segments into a larger network and forwards packets to the appropriate segment.

6.13   What is a DBMS

Electronic information is stored in a database management system (DBMS). Think of this as an electronic filing cabinet and a super–file clerk all rolled up in one.

6.14　What is encryption?

Encryption is a process of converting information to a meaningless series of letters and numbers that can be stored or transmitted with little chance of anyone who doesn't have the cipher being able to convert it back to readable information

6.15　What is a key?

At the heart of the conversion process is a mathematical formula that uses a value called a key to transform meaningful information into meaningless information (encryption) and meaningless information to meaningful information (decipher).

6.16　What is a privacy filter?

A privacy filter prevents anyone except the person in front of the computer from clearly seeing the image on the screen.

6.17　What is the function of an end user services group within the healthcare facility's IT department?

The end user services group is responsible for the computer equipment on the unit and in the offices. This group is called whenever anything goes wrong with the workstation or if new equipment needs to be ordered.

6.18　What is the function of the network group within the healthcare facility's IT department?

The network group is responsible for the hardware and software that is necessary to send and receive information over the computer network.

6.19　What is the function of the applications group within the healthcare facility's IT department?

The applications group is in control of specialty programs such as the charting programs that run on all computers in the healthcare facility. They are the in-house experts called for assistance using that program.

6.20　What is the function of the administration group within the healthcare facility's IT department?

The administration group sets the IT strategies and policies for the healthcare facility and oversees the operation of the other four groups within the IT division.

6.21　Who can receive Wi-Fi information within a healthcare facility?

Any receiver tuned to the Wi-Fi's frequency can receive the signal, but only authorized receivers can understand the data that are being transmitted. All data are encrypted before being transmitted. Only a receiver with the proper cipher can decipher the data, and this protects the data from eavesdropping computer devices that connect to Wi-Fi.

6.22　How can information on the workstation screen be protected when the person leaves the workstation?

It is common for the workstation to automatically erase information from the screen and log out the user after a period of time has passed to assure that the information remains secure. This reduces the risk that patient information can be viewed on the screen after the user walks away from the workstation or that another person can use the workstation while the user is still logged in.

6.23   What happens to information that is stored in the workstation's memory?

Information stored in memory is erased automatically when the workstation is turned off.

6.24   How are charting software the same yet different?

A charting program lets the healthcare provider use the computer to record, retrieve, edit, and print a patient's chart. There are many different kinds of charting programs available, all of which are used to electronically chart patient information; however each does so in a slightly different way.

6.25   What is an operating system?

A special group of computer programs called an operating system enables a workstation to process charting information.

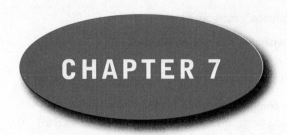

CHAPTER 7

Charting Software

7.1   Definition

Charting software is similar to the software used on a personal or home computer. It transforms the computer into a tool to document a patient's health electronically and shares patient information with the healthcare team no matter where they are located.

Charting software eliminates:

- Clumsy loose-leaf binders
- Scratchy handwriting that is difficult to decipher
- Difficulties sharing patient information

7.2   Different Charting Software

There isn't just one charting program used by every healthcare facility. Each facility chooses charting software from among several manufacturers who are prominent in the field.

This is similar to word processing software. Everyone with a computer has word processing software, however not everyone uses Microsoft Word word processing software. As with different word processing software, different charting software is similar yet different. Each works basically the same way. Regardless of the manufacturer of the charting software, the healthcare provider will be able to:

- Select a patient from a list of his or her patients
- Display the patient's electronic chart including the MAR (medication administration record), labs, and medical orders
- Update the chart with an assessment of the patient
- Enter orders
- Order labs

Charting software has push buttons, drop-down lists, scrolling lists, text boxes, and other objects that are used in Microsoft Word, Excel, Windows, and other software.

Double clicking a patient's name that appears on a list of patients displays that patient's chart because the healthcare provider selected information from a list in other software such as a document to open in Word. Clicking a push button labeled Find starts a search for his or her patients.

Charting software differs from manufacturer to manufacturer in the way the chart is organized and the way information is entered and displayed. The best way to learn to use any charting software is to first find out how the charting software is organized and how to use its features.

7.3   Getting Started

The folks at McKesson, a leading manufacturer of charting software, agreed to let us walk through how to use their software as a way to get acquainted with electronic charting. This chapter shows how McKesson's software is organized and various ways to find a patient's chart. The remaining chapters show how to enter an assessment of the patient, enter orders, review the MAR, and document other common tasks.

7.3.1   Logging In

A log-in process is used to log into the healthcare facility's computer. A log-in screen prompts the user to enter his or her ID and password, which is assigned to each member of the healthcare team by the IT department.

This ID is granted rights to access the healthcare facility's computerized charting software. Think of a right as a permission. This means anyone using this ID has the same rights because the computer thinks that's who is logged in. Therefore it is important that the healthcare provider does not share his ID and password with anyone.

Depending on the healthcare provider's responsibilities and the policies of the healthcare facility, he is granted rights to various features of the software.

With charting software the healthcare provider might be granted rights to:

- Access the chart of some or all patients

- Update some or all components of the chart

- Delete information from the chart

- Reassign patients

- Enter orders or specific types of orders

- Access reports

The nurse might see different features on the screen than her supervisor sees because each has rights to different features of the software. For example, the nurse may see a list of only her patients while the supervisor sees a list of all patients in the unit.

7.3.1.1   The Password

The healthcare provider will be asked to change his password the first time he logs in. He can pick his own password, however some healthcare facilities set minimum requirements for a password such as its length; a combination of characters, numbers, and punctuation; and the ease in which the password can be guessed or hacked. The healthcare provider alone knows this password.

The healthcare provider may also be asked to provide a question and answer to be used in case of a forgotten password. The question might be what school he attended. The answer is the name of his school. If he forgets his password, he clicks the reminder button on the log-in screen. The question is displayed and he is prompted to enter the answer. If correct, his password is emailed to him.

The healthcare facility may require the healthcare provider to contact the IT department for a forgotten password rather than letting the user click a password reminder button on the log-in screen. The IT department then resets the password and emails it to the user. The healthcare provider will then be required to change the password the next time she logs in. The IT department is not privy to the new password.

7.3.1.2 Frequent Log-Ins

Expect to be required to log in frequently. Healthcare facilities usually have a policy requiring automatic log-outs if the computer sits idle for a few minutes. The assumption is that the healthcare provider walked away from the computer without logging off and a patient's information may be displayed on the screen.

The amount of time that needs to expire prior to being logged out is determined by the IT department. The healthcare provider can easily regain access by entering her ID and password into the log-in screen.

Moving the mouse every so often when spending a long time reading the screen can prevent the automatic log-out.

7.3.2 The Log

The healthcare provider's activities on the computer are probably recorded in an electronic log. An entry is made at log-in and log-out. Entries might contain what software is used; what features of the software are used and what charts are viewed or changed. Nearly everything might be tracked.

Each log entry contains the user's ID; date and time that he or she gained access; the date and time access was terminated; the unique ID of the computer used; and other specific information about the user's activities.

The IT department refers to these entries whenever there is suspicion that the healthcare policy was violated. From time to time the healthcare facility and regulatory agencies may audit the log to assure compliance with policies and regulation.

The healthcare provider should assume that everything he or she does using the healthcare facility's computers is being monitored, including surfing the Internet.

7.4 The Chart Begins

Charting software is used to store general information about the patient such as name, address, insurance carrier, and the patient's medical information.

The patient's chart begins when the admissions staff enters the patient's general information when the patient is admitted to the healthcare facility. This information is stored in a central database. Each member of the healthcare team electronically retrieves it at the click of the mouse and updates the patient's chart to reflect his or her assessment and treatment plan.

If the patient was previously admitted to the healthcare facility, then the patient's information already exist in the database. The admissions staff and the patient's healthcare team then retrieve and update the information based on the patient's current condition.

7.5 Locating a Patient's Chart

There are a number of ways to find a patient's chart using charting software, the easiest of which is to select the patient from a list. Charting software displays a list of patients who are admitted to the unit. This list is called a census.

The list appears in a table (Figure 7.1) similar in appearance to a spreadsheet where each row represents a patient and columns contain key information about the patient such as:

Notify	Last	First	Dept	Rm/Bed	Diagnosis	Gen...	MRN
0	DANIELS	MELANIE	24N	2400-1	(W) ABDOMINAL PAIN UNSPEC...	F	000001055
1	EDGAR	MARNIE	24N	2400-2	(W) LUMP OR MASS IN BREAS...	F	000001054
2	FREMONT	LISA CAROL	24N	2401-1	(W) PATHOLOGIC FX,UNSPEC...	F	000001060
3	CRANE	LILA	24N	2402-1	(W) OTALGIA NOS (388.70)	F	000001056
4	TYLER	BLANCHE	24N	2402-2	(W) NEUROTIC DEPRESSION (...	F	000001065
5	DEVEREAUX	ANDRE	24N	2403-1	(W) CHEST PAIN NOS (786.50)	M	000001052
6	BLANEY	RICHARD	24N	2403-2	(W) FEVER (780.6)	M	000001051
7	LUMLEY	GEORGE	24N	2404-1	(W) CHEST PAIN NOS (786.50)	M	000001050
8	OACKLEY	CHARLIE	24N	2406-1	(W) GASTROINTEST HEMORR...	M	000001061
9	JEFFRIES	JEFF LB	24N	2407-2	(W) FLU W RESP MANIFEST N...	M	000001059

Figure 7.1

- Notify

- Last name

- First name

- Department

- Room/bed

- Diagnosis

- Gender

- Medical record number

Patients are sorted by information in one or more columns. The charting software determines the default sort order, which in McKesson's case is by room and bed. It is easy to re-sort the list by clicking the column name to be sorted. For example, clicking the Last column sorts the list by the patient's last name (Figure 7.2).

Notice that the list has the same scroll bar that is found on other Windows software. Click the up and down arrows to scroll incrementally. Drag the scroll bar to move quickly through the list. Click the top and bottom icons (below the down arrow) to jump to the top and bottom of the list.

7.5.1 Filtering the List

Having the full list of patients available is handy when the healthcare provider is covering a patient for another member of the healthcare team. By double clicking the patient's name, the charting software displays the patient's chart on the screen.

The healthcare provider will probably want to see some, but not all, patients' names based on the task that is being performed. This is possible by filtering the list to only patients that the healthcare provider needs to see.

Above the table is a row of empty boxes, one for each column. Enter a value in the box and the charting software displays patients who have that value. Suppose the healthcare provider is assigned to department 24N and he wants to see a list of patients who are admitted to that department. By entering the 24N in the empty box above the Dept. column, only those patients in department 24N are displayed on the screen (Figure 7.3).

Some empty boxes have drop-down lists. A drop-down list shows valid entries such as department and gender values. It is only possible to pick a value from the list provided in the drop-down list. It is not possible to enter a value that is not on the list. Other empty boxes such as last name and first name can accept any value.

7.5.2 More Filtering

Whether the healthcare provider is viewing a list of all the patients or just her own patients, she can use predefined filters to reduce the list to a specific category of patient. The categories can differ depending on the charting software; some charting software programs enable the healthcare facility to create their own categories.

For example, McKesson's charting software has three categories called type, status, and facility. Type describes if the patient is an inpatient, emergency, outpatient, in and out patient, or obstetrics patient. Status is defined as active, discharged, pre-admit, and expired. The facilities category identifies the division of the healthcare that is caring for the patient such as Link 3 East (the east wing of the third floor in the Link Building).

Categories are selected by picking the category from a drop-down box located at the bottom of the list. Clicking the Type down arrow displays the drop-down list and then clicking Inpatient displays a list of all inpatients (Figure 7.4).

Notify	Last	/	First	Dept.	Rm/Bed	Diagnosis		Gen...	MRN
0	ARMSTRONG		MICHAEL	24N	2410-1	(W) CHEST PAIN NOS (786.50)		M	000001053
1	BLANEY		RICHARD	24N	2403-2	(W) FEVER (780.6)		M	000001051
2	CHILDRESS		ROBERT	24N	2408-1	(W) BRONCHITIS NOS (490), (F...		M	000001149
3	CRANE		LILA	24N	2402-1	(W) OTALGIA NOS (388.70)		F	000001056
4	DANIELS		MELANIE	24N	2400-1	(W) ABDOMINAL PAIN UNSPEC...		F	000001055
5	DEVEREAUX		ANDRE	24N	2403-1	(W) CHEST PAIN NOS (786.50)		M	000001052
6	EDGAR		MARNIE	24N	2400-2	(W) LUMP OR MASS IN BREAS...		F	000001054
7	EVERGUARD		ELIZABETH	24N	2409-1	(W) TACHYCARDIA NOS (785.0)		F	000001121
8	FREMONT		LISA CAROL	24N	2401-1	(W) PATHOLOGIC FX/UNSPEC...		F	000001060
9	JEFFRIES		JEFF LB	24N	2407-2	(W) FLU W RESP MANIFEST N...		M	000001059

Figure 7.2

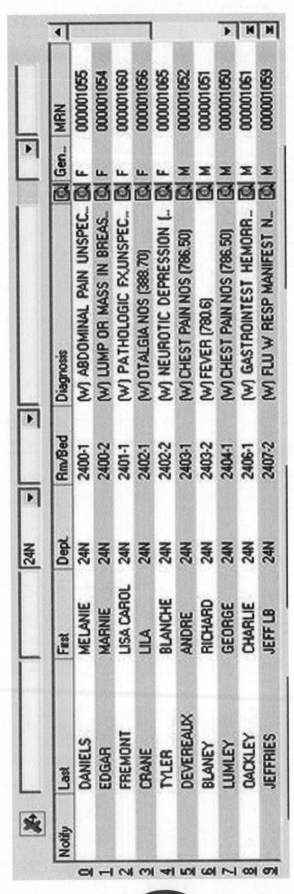

Figure 7.3

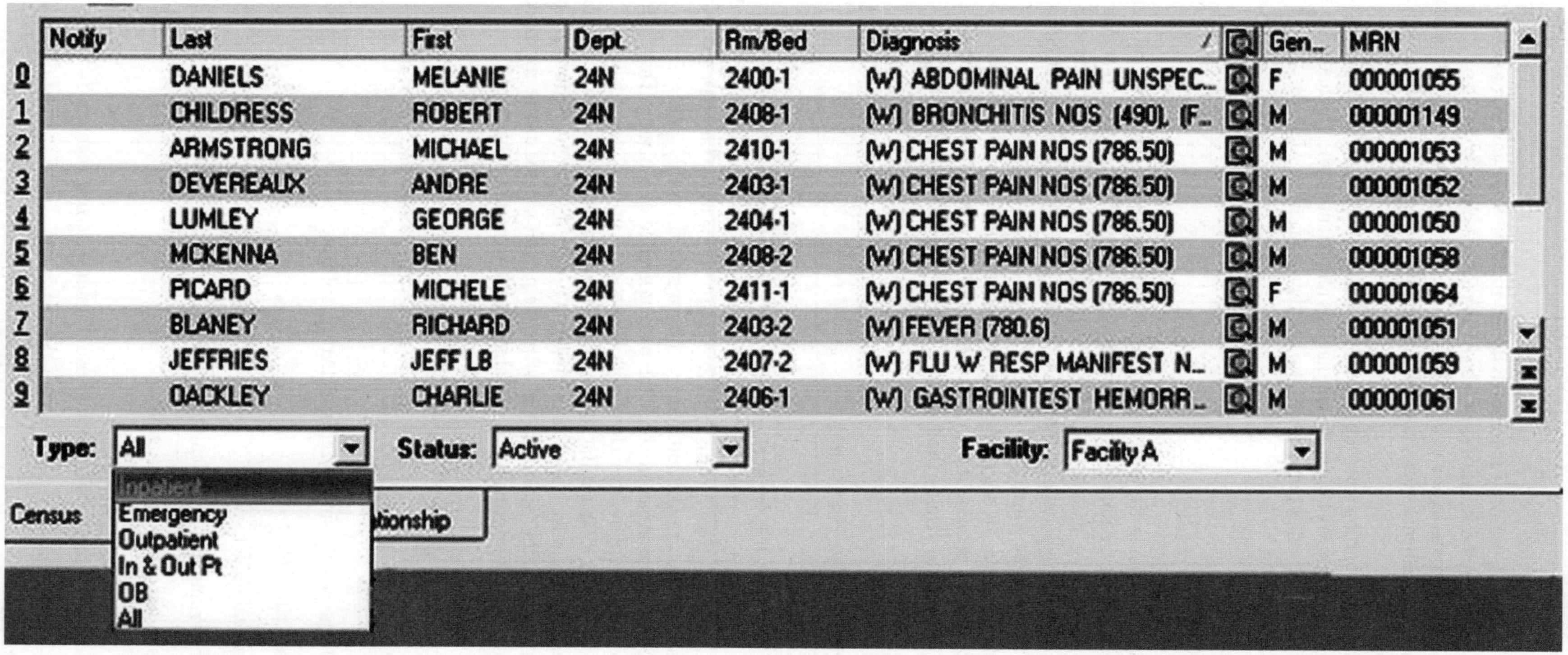

	Notify	Last	First	Dept.	Rm/Bed	Diagnosis		Gen...	MRN
0		DANIELS	MELANIE	24N	2400-1	(W) ABDOMINAL PAIN UNSPEC...		F	000001055
1		CHILDRESS	ROBERT	24N	2408-1	(W) BRONCHITIS NOS (490), (F...		M	000001149
2		ARMSTRONG	MICHAEL	24N	2410-1	(W) CHEST PAIN NOS (786.50)		M	000001053
3		DEVEREAUX	ANDRE	24N	2403-1	(W) CHEST PAIN NOS (786.50)		M	000001052
4		LUMLEY	GEORGE	24N	2404-1	(W) CHEST PAIN NOS (786.50)		M	000001050
5		MCKENNA	BEN	24N	2408-2	(W) CHEST PAIN NOS (786.50)		M	000001058
6		PICARD	MICHELE	24N	2411-1	(W) CHEST PAIN NOS (786.50)		F	000001064
7		BLANEY	RICHARD	24N	2403-2	(W) FEVER (780.6)		M	000001051
8		JEFFRIES	JEFF LB	24N	2407-2	(W) FLU W RESP MANIFEST N...		M	000001059
9		OACKLEY	CHARLIE	24N	2406-1	(W) GASTROINTEST HEMORR...		M	000001061

Type: All
Inpatient
Emergency
Outpatient
In & Out Pt
OB
All
Status: Active
Facility: Facility A
Census
...tionship

Figure 7.4

7.5.3   Find a Patient

Typically, the nurse will want to see only patients assigned to him by the nurse manager. The McKesson's charting software does this when the Relationship tab (Figure 7.5) is clicked.

Other charting software programs have a comparable feature. The relationship is both primary and secondary (covering) responsibility for the patient as determined by the nurse manager. The charting software removes from the list all except your patients.

You might wonder how the charting software knows which patients are assigned to you. Staffing assignments are made using a management feature of the software that lists all patients in the unit and enables the nurse manager to assign each to a nurse and other members of the healthcare team.

7.5.4   Partial Matches

The healthcare provider may not know the correct spelling of a patient's name. However, by entering a few letters of the patient's name and clicking the Find button, the charting software finds patients that match.

Suppose that last name begins with *Jeff*. Enter these letters in the empty box over the Last column and McKesson's charting software displays possible matches (Figure 7.6) on the list. Of course, the healthcare provider will still need to verify the patient.

In this example, McKesson's charting software displays all charts for the patient. Notice that the first row is missing a discharge date because the patient is currently admitted to the unit. Subsequent rows have the discharge date and are used to display the patient's charts from previous admissions.

7.6   Displaying the Patient's Chart

Once the patient is located on the list, the next step is to open the patient's chart on the screen by selecting the patient. Double click the row containing the patient's name and the charting software presents the patient's chart.

Figure 7.7 is the McKesson's chart for Elisabeth Everguard. At the top of the chart above the patient's name is a menu of features used to help analyze and manage information about this patient.

Below, the menu contains information about the patient needed at a glance. This includes the patient's account number and medical record number along with the patient's primary diagnosis.

Tabs divide the chart into sections similar to tabs in a ring-binder chart. Clicking the tab opens the corresponding section of the chart where the nurse can review and update the patient's information.

By default the chart opens to the vital signs tab where the patient's status can be reviewed quickly. How to enter vital signs and other patient information is explained in the remaining chapters.

Solved Problems

7.1   What are the advantages of using electronic charting software?

Charting software eliminates:

- Clumsy loose-leaf binder

- Scratchy handwriting that is difficult to decipher

- Difficulties sharing patient information

7.2   Why is it that healthcare facilities frequently use different charting software?

Each healthcare facility selects a software manufacturer whose product provides the most cost-effective solutions.

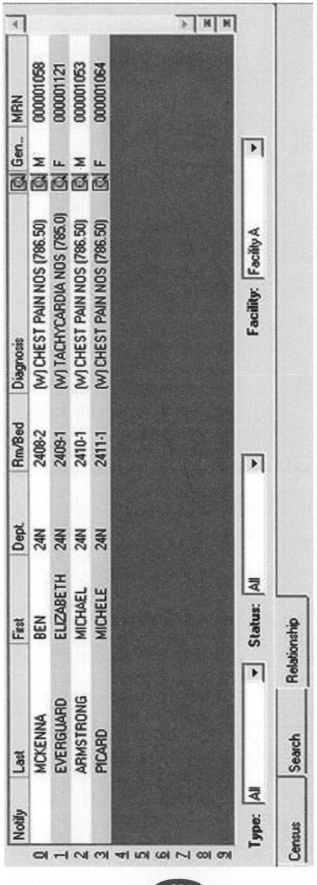

Figure 7.5

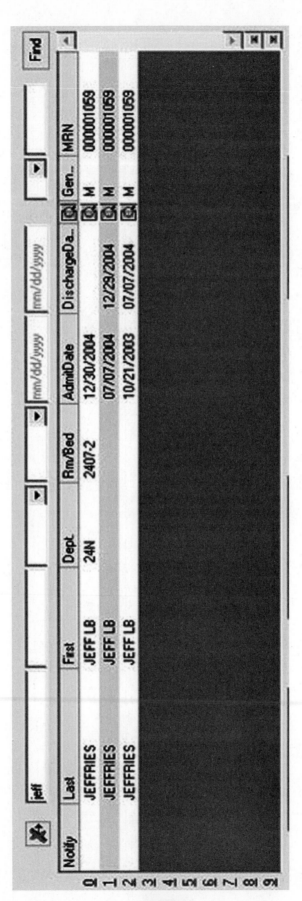

Figure 7.6

92

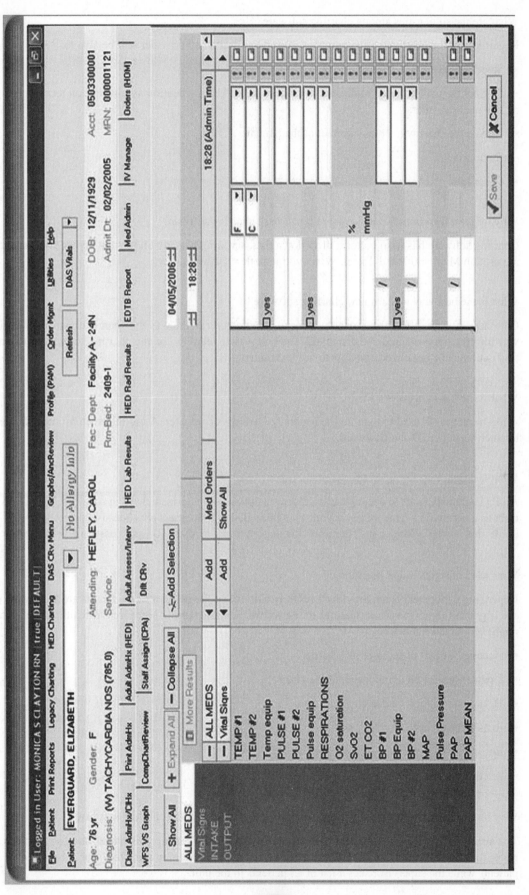

Figure 7.7

7.3   What are the similarities among charting software?

Regardless of the charting software manufacturer, the healthcare provider will be able to:

- Select a patient from a list of patients

- Display the patient's electronic chart including the MAR (medication administration record), labs, and medical orders

- Update the chart with an assessment of the patient

- Enter orders

- Order labs

7.4   Why might it be relatively easy to learn how to use charting software?

Charting software has push buttons, drop-down lists, scrolling lists, text boxes, and other objects that are used in Microsoft Word, Excel, Windows, and other software.

7.5   What is the best way to learn new charting software?

Charting software differs from manufacturer to manufacturer in the way the chart is organized and the way information is entered and displayed. The best way to learn to use any charting software is to first find out how it is organized and how to use its features.

7.6   What is the log-in process?

A log-in process is used to log into the healthcare facility's computer. A log-in screen prompts the user to enter his or her ID and password.

7.7   What is a right?

An ID is granted rights to access the healthcare facility's computerized charting software. Think of a right as a permission. This means anyone using this ID has the same rights because the computer thinks that is who is logged in. Therefore it is important not to share IDs and passwords with anyone.

7.8   What kind of rights might be granted?

Depending on the healthcare provider's responsibilities and the policies of the healthcare facility, he or she is granted rights to various features of the software. With charting software the healthcare provider might be granted rights to:

- Access the chart of some or all patients

- Update some or all components of the chart

- Delete information from a chart

- Reassign patients

- Enter orders or specific types of orders

- Access reports

7.9   Why might the nurse and the supervisor see different features on the charting software?

The nurse might see different features on the screen than his or her supervisor sees because each has rights to different features of the software. For example, the nurse may see a list of only his or her patients while the supervisor sees a list of all patients in the unit.

7.10   Why might a healthcare provider be asked to supply a question and its answer when setting up his password?

He may be asked to provide a question and answer to be used for a forgotten password. The question might be what school did you attend. The answer is the name of his school. If he forgets his password, he can click the reminder button on the log-in screen. The question is displayed and he is prompted to enter the answer. If answered correctly, his password is emailed to him.

7.11   What will the IT department do in the case of a forgotten password?

The IT department resets the password and emails it to the user. The password must be changed the next time the user logs in.

7.12   Does the IT department know each password?

No. The IT department can only reset a password and require that the new temporary password be changed at the next log-in.

7.13   Why might a user be logged off the computer if the computer sits idle for a few minutes?

The assumption is that the healthcare provider walked away from the computer without logging off and probably left a patient's information displayed on the screen.

7.14   Who determines the amount of time that needs to expire before being logged out?

The amount of time that needs to expire prior to being logged out is determined by the IT department.

7.15   What is a log?

Activities on the computer are probably recorded in an electronic log.

7.16   What might be recorded in a log?

An entry is made when a user logs in and when he or she logs out. Entries might contain what software is used; what features of the software are used; and what charts are viewed or changed. Nearly everything the user does might be tracked.

7.17   Why is an electronic log maintained?

The IT department refers to these entries whenever there is suspicion that the healthcare policy was violated. From time to time the healthcare facility and regulatory agencies may audit the log to assure compliance with policies and regulation.

7.18   When does the electronic chart begin?

The patient's chart begins when the admissions staff enters the patient's general information when the patient is admitted to the healthcare facility.

7.19   Where is patient information stored?

Patient information is stored in a central database.

7.20   What might occur if the patient was previously admitted to the hospital?

If the patient was previously admitted to the healthcare facility, then the patient's information already exists in the database. The admissions staff and the patient's healthcare team then retrieve and update the information based on the patient's current condition.

7.21   What is the most common way of finding a patient's chart for a patient who is on a unit?

There are a number of ways to find a patient's chart using charting software, the easiest of which is to select the patient from a list. Charting software displays a list of patients who are admitted to the unit called a census.

7.22   What might you expect to see on a list of patients?

- Last name
- First name
- Department
- Room/bed
- Diagnosis
- Gender
- Medical record number

7.23   How might you change the order of patients?

Patients are sorted by information in one or more columns. The charting software determines the default sort order, which in McKesson's case is by room and bed. It is easy to re-sort the list by clicking the column name to be sorted.

7.24   What is a filter?

A filter is a feature of charting software that reduces a list of patients to patients that meet the filter criteria.

7.25   What is a partial match?

A partial match is a feature of charting software that enables locating a patient without knowing the correct spelling of the patient's name. Enter the first few letters of the patient's name and the charting software will find patients who match the criteria.

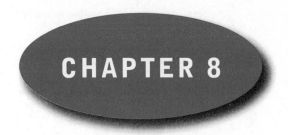

CHAPTER 8

Basic Electronic Charting

8.1 Definition

Three basic nursing routines include actions to carry out medical orders, monitor vital signs, and measure intake and output. There are electronic charts available to assist the nurse performing these routines.

8.2 To-Do List

Patients are assigned to each nurse by the charge nurse using the charting software. After report, the nurse needs to know orders scheduled for each patient. After logging into the electronic charting system, assigned patients are automatically displayed on the opening screen showing the patient's name, medical record number, and a to-do list of pending orders, depending on the electronic charting system that is used in the healthcare facility.

Figure 8.1 shows the to-do list of activities presented in the McKesson software. Activities include scheduled medication, assessment, and labs.

Each patient is identified on a row by the patient's name, unit, room/bed number, and medical record number. The entry also contains the name of an activity called Ordered Item and practitioner's order number enabling the nurse to quickly trace the activity back to the original practitioner's order. Rows containing patient information are identified by alternating bands of color making it easy to distinguish patients on the list.

In addition, there is information displayed that is needed to perform the activity. For example, patient Lila Crane is scheduled to receive Fluorouracil/Dextrose 5 percent at 10 a.m. IV. The dose is 489 mg/1,000 ml at a rate of 42 ml/hr.

Activities that must be performed immediately are marked as Stat and highlighted in red providing a clear visual indication and drawing the nurse's attention to the activity.

Each entry contains the date and time when the activity is scheduled. The Status column indicates Scheduled or Overdue. Schedule means the activity is planned but not as yet due to be performed. The electronic charting software will highlight Schedule status when the activity is currently due. Past due activities are marked as Overdue indicating that the scheduled date and time for the activity has passed.

At the top of the screen is a filter bar. The filter bar is used to set criteria for displaying patient information. The left corner of the filter bar contains four radio buttons—each a classification of order. The number alongside each classification is the number of activities within the classification.

Overdues (13)　Changes (41)　Current shift
To Do (21)　Active (69)　Time range

From: 05/22/06　09:39　To: 05/22/06　21:45

Refresh　Details

Patient Name	Scheduled	Group	Status	Ordered Item	Dose/Duration	Route	Prty Freq (Rate)	Order #'s	Comm
CRANE, LILA	05/22 10:00	IVS	Scheduled	FLUOROURACIL/DEXTROSE 5%	489 MG/1000 ML	IV	42 ml/hr	7544 (1)	CYTO
24N 2402-1 MRN:000001058	05/22 10:40	NSG	Overdue	ASSESS FOR CHEST PAIN			TODAY ONCE	2323858	
	05/22 10:50	LAB	Overdue	COMPLETE BLOOD COUNT			STAT STAT	2323866	
	05/22 17:00	LAB	Scheduled	COMPLETE BLOOD COUNT			ROUTINE ONCE	2323862	
TYLER, BLANCHE	05/22 12:00	DTY	Overdue	LOW TRIGLYCERIDE			DTY TIMED MEALS	2323667	
24N 2402-2 MRN:000001064	05/22 17:00	DTY	Scheduled	LOW TRIGLYCERIDE			DTY TIMED MEALS	2323668	
DEVEREAUX, ANDRE	05/22 10:39	NSG	Overdue	ASSESS FOR CHEST PAIN	1 Occurrence		TODAY ONCE	2323818	
24N 2403-1 MRN:000001057	05/22 17:00	LAB	Scheduled	COMPLETE BLOOD COUNT	1 Occurrence		ROUTINE ONCE	2323823	
JEFFRIES, JEFF LB	05/22 10:40	LAB	Overdue	COMPLETE BLOOD COUNT	1 Occurrence		TODAY ONCE	2323813	
24N 2407-2 MRN:000001059		NSG	Overdue	ASSESS FOR CHEST PAIN	1 Occurrence		TODAY ONCE	2323811	
CHILDRESS, ROBERT	05/22 10:00	IVS	Scheduled	POTASSIUM PHOSPHATE DIBASIC/D5W	.5 MMOLE/1000 ML	IV	100 ml/hr	7551 (2)	
24N 2408-1 MRN:000001149	05/22 10:38	NSG	Overdue	ASSESS FOR CHEST PAIN	1 Occurrence		ROUTINE ONCE	2323804	
	05/22 17:00	LAB	Scheduled	COMPLETE BLOOD COUNT	1 Occurrence		ROUTINE ONCE	2323809	
EVERGUARD, ELIZABETH	05/22 10:41	NSG	Overdue	ASSESS FOR CHEST PAIN	1 Occurrence		TODAY ONCE	2323832	
24N 2409-1 MRN:000001127	05/22 12:00	DTY	Overdue	CARDIAC DIET			DTY TIMED MEALS	2323870	
	05/22 17:00	DTY	Scheduled	CARDIAC DIET			DTY TIMED MEALS	2323671	
		LAB	Scheduled	COMPLETE BLOOD COUNT	1 Occurrence		ROUTINE ONCE	2323837	
KENDALL, EVE	05/22 10:40	NSG	Overdue	ASSESS FOR CHEST PAIN	1 Occurrence		ROUTINE ONCE	2323825	
24N 2413-2 MRN:000001063	05/22 17:00	LAB	Scheduled	CBC (Complete Blood Count)	1 Occurrence		ROUTINE ONCE	2323830	
NEWTON, CHARLIE	05/22 10:40	NSG	Overdue	ASSESS FOR CHEST PAIN	1 Occurrence		ROUTINE ONCE	2323839	
24N 2414-2 MRN:000001061	05/22 17:00	LAB	Scheduled	COMPLETE BLOOD COUNT	1 Occurrence		ROUTINE 012H	2323844	

Figure 8.1

In Figure 8.1, there are 13 overdue activities. Selecting the Overdues radio button causes the electronic charting system to display only overdue activities. All other activities are filtered from the display. There are 21 To Do activities. These include scheduled and overdue activities. The To Do radio button is selected in this example. Changes are activities that have changed, which are typically activities that are completed and revised orders. There are 41 Changes activities indicated but not shown in this example.

Active are activities that have been scheduled for now and in the future. There are 69 activities in the Active category. Typically, the nurse will want to view a subset of Active activities based on a specified date and time. Activities are displayed based on one of two filters. These are Current shift and Time range. Current shift means that only activities that are either scheduled for the current shift or are overdue from a previous shift are displayed. A shift is defined in the electronic charting software by an administrator. The electronic charting software uses the computer's clock to identify the current date and time and therefore knows activities that fall within the current shift.

Alternatively, a date and time range can be entered into the filter bar enabling the nurse to determine date and time of activities to display. In this example, on Active activities scheduled between 5/22/06 at 9:39 and 5/22/06 at 21:45 are displayed.

Once the filter criteria are set, the Refresh button is selected to apply the filter to the Active activities. Some electronic charting software may automatically refresh activities whenever a filter is changed, however don't assume that the list of activities is refreshed. Always verify that information on the screen complies with the filter requirements.

If more information about the order is needed, then highlight the order and select the Details button to display full information about the order. Double clicking the order will also display detail information about the order without having to select the Details button. The detail screen is also where the activity is updated, such as indicating that the order was carried out.

8.3 Vital Signs

The vital signs section of the McKesson's charting software is organized into groups called classes that appear in the left column and are referred to as the navigation panel. The classifications are ALL MEDS, VITAL SIGNS, I&O SUMMARY, INTAKE, and OUTPUT. Double clicking a classification with the mouse opens the classification in either Review Mode or Chart Mode, which lets the healthcare provider enter new vital signs into the chart.

Review Mode displays previous entries such as vital signs shown in Figure 8.2. Use the right scroll bar to scroll down and up the list of vital signs and use the horizontal scroll bar at the bottom of the screen to scroll right or left to see a history of the patient's vital signs.

Vital signs that are beyond the normal range are highlighted in red. Although the electronic charting software automatically uses widely accepted normal ranges the administrator of the charting software can modify these ranges based on the policies of the healthcare facility.

8.3.1 Entering Vital Signs

The nurse clicks the Chart button (see Figure 8.2) to enter the Chart Mode and enter new vital signs for the patient. The charting software opens a screen where the nurse can enter a new set of vital signs, and it automatically enters the date and time based on the current date and time.

A common problem is that the current time is not the time when vital signs are taken—it is the time when the nurse enters vital signs into the charting software. It is critical that the date and time reflect when the vital signs are taken and not the date and time when vital signs are entered. There are scroll arrows that you can use to change it to the correct date and time.

Double clicking the name of the vital sign in the Vital Signs column opens an area of the chart where new values can be entered. The nurse can enter a value or select a value from a drop-down list depending on the nature of the vital sign that he is entering into the chart.

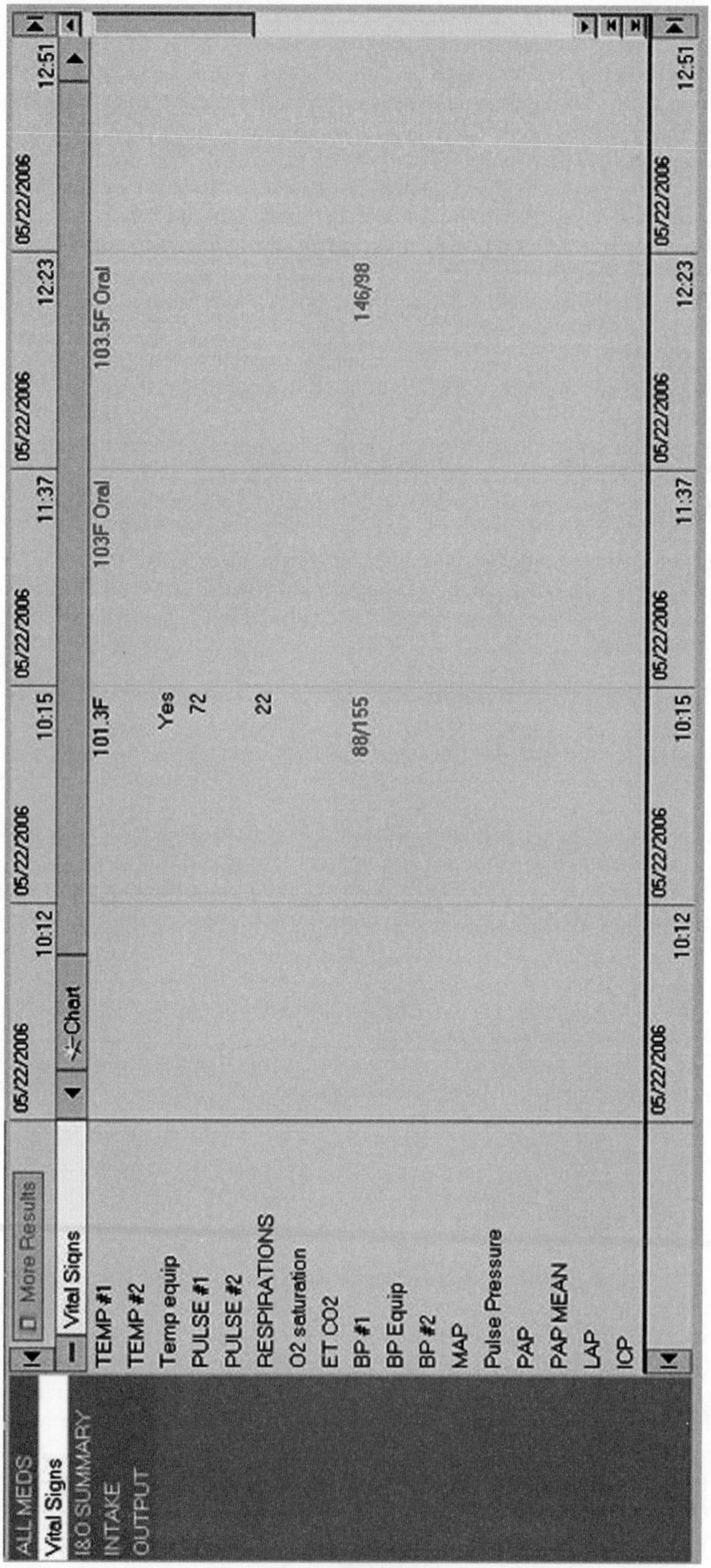
ALL MEDS
Vital Signs
I&O SUMMARY
INTAKE
OUTPUT
More Results
Vital Signs
Chart
05/22/2006 10:12
05/22/2006 10:15
05/22/2006 11:37
05/22/2006 12:23
05/22/2006 12:51
TEMP #1
TEMP #2
Temp equip
PULSE #1
PULSE #2
RESPIRATIONS
O2 saturation
ET CO2
BP #1
BP Equip
BP #2
MAP
Pulse Pressure
PAP
PAP MEAN
LAP
ICP
101.3F
Yes
72
22
88/155
103F Oral
103.5F Oral
146/98

Figure 8.2

Let's say that the nurse is entering the patient's temperature for the second time in the day. Clicking TEMP #2 opens the temperature row in the chart. The nurse types "103" and then opens the next drop-down list to select "F" for Fahrenheit. (The other option is Celsius.) Then he selects the last drop-down list box in that row to identify how the temperature was taken (Figure 8.3).

Depending on the charting software, the nurse is also able to select default values for drop-down lists based on common practice in that healthcare facility. For example, a healthcare facility might always use Fahrenheit and Tympanic. These can be designated as default settings and will appear in the box. This saves times when entering vital signs. Some charting software requires that these default settings be made for each patient, usually the first time vital signs are entered. Other charting software will enable the administrator of the charting software to establish default settings for all patients.

8.3.2   Red Flag the Vital Signs

When a vital sign is significant the nurse calls attention to it by setting a red flag and entering a comment. McKesson's charting software uses an exclamation mark as the red flag. Click the exclamation mark found at the right of the vital sign and the charting software displays the exclamation mark in red. Click the exclamation mark a second time to turn off the flag.

8.4   Comments

The exclamation mark can be used to call the attention of other members of the patient's healthcare team throughout the electronic chart for any significant change, not just for vital signs. In addition, the nurse can explain concerns by entering a comment into the electronic chart.

Take the patient's weight as an example. The patient's weight is entered into the computerized chart similar to the method for temperature in that the nurse enters the weight and corresponding metric such as ounces, kilograms, milligram, or grams. Suppose the weight changed significantly. This wouldn't be obvious even if the exclamation flag is turned on. The question is, what is the significance?

Charting software enables the healthcare provider to write a note explaining the significance. The note section is opened by clicking an icon on the computerized chart. With McKesson's charting software, the icon to the right of the exclamation mark is clicked. This opens a text box where up to 255 characters may be entered. In the weight example, the nurse might write "Lost 2 lb in 2 days" (Figure 8.4).

8.5   Charting I&O

Intake and output are measured and recorded in a patient's chart. A major advantage of electronic charting over paper charts is that the charting software automatically performs calculations as long as intake and output amounts are entered correctly.

Select I&O SUMMARY class in the left navigation panel (Figure 8.5) to display total intake, total output, and the net value for each day and time that is charged. Scrolling to the left and right displays results for additional days and time.

Items are entered as volume or occurrences. A volume is a measurable amount of fluid and is measured in milliliters. An occurrence is fluid that is not measurable, such as an apple. Only volume is included in the I&O calculation.

Below the summary section is an itemized list of intake and output charted. In this example, the nurse recorded the patient's intake at 10:12 on 5/22/2006 to be 50 ml of oral fluids, 8 ml of Ensure for a total intake of 58 ml. The patient's urine output was 25 ml for a total output of 25 ml.

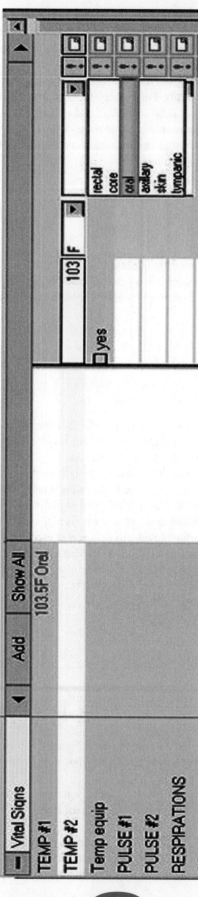

Figure 8.3

102

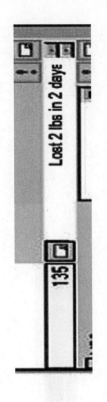

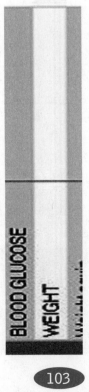

Figure 8.4

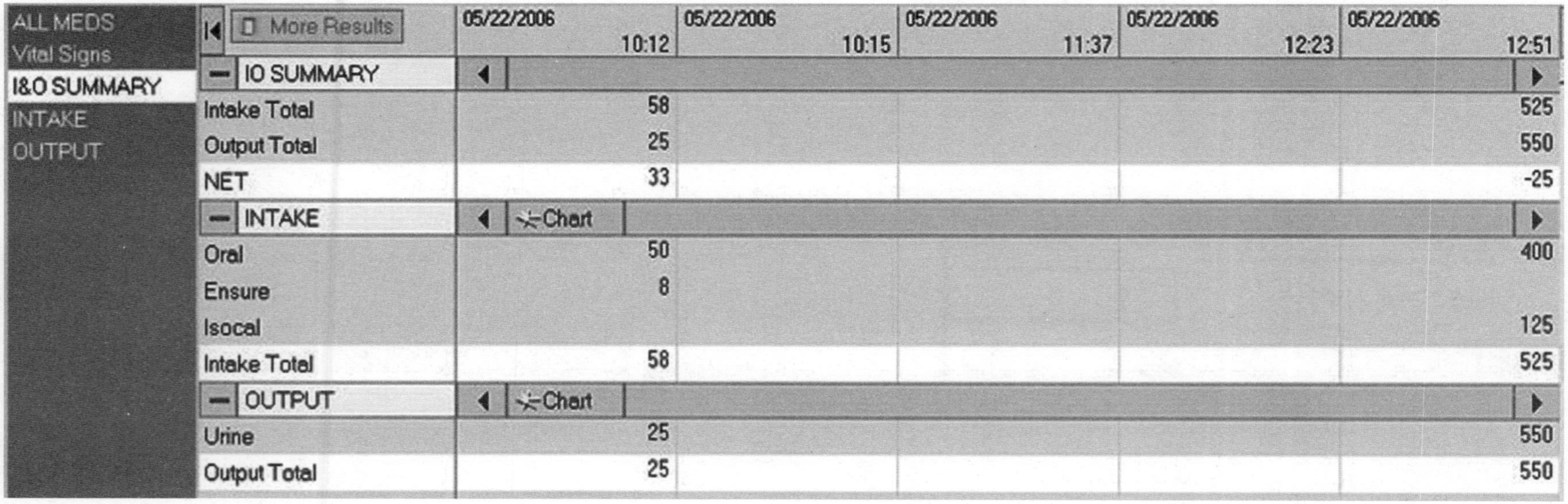

	05/22/2006 10:12	05/22/2006 10:15	05/22/2006 11:37	05/22/2006 12:23	05/22/2006 12:51
More Results					
— IO SUMMARY					
Intake Total	58				525
Output Total	25				550
NET	33				-25
— INTAKE	Chart				
Oral	50				400
Ensure	8				
Isocal					125
Intake Total	58				525
— OUTPUT	Chart				
Urine	25				550
Output Total	25				550

ALL MEDS
Vital Signs
I&O SUMMARY
INTAKE
OUTPUT

Figure 8.5

104

8.5.1   Entering I&O

Entering intake and output values is similar to entering vital signs into the chart. Click the appropriate class (Intake or Output) in the navigation bar to display the page. The page contains a list of items that the healthcare facility wants measured. Double click the item and the charting software opens an area where the nurse can enter a value or select the Chart button. A drop-down list displays common items for intake and output. The administrator of the charting software typically is able to insert and remove items in drop-down lists and order items on the list in a most-used order, which speeds entering charting information.

8.6   Reviewing the Entry

Click the Save button after updating the patient's chart. The Save button displays the review page (Figure 8.6) and the entries. Each entry may be reviewed before the information is saved to the patient's chart.

In this example, the temperature and weight are displayed. The exclamation is set to red indicating there is a significant result that the nurse wants others on the healthcare team to review. Likewise, there is a note written about a change in the patient's weight (losing two pounds in two days).

There are four choices each displayed as buttons at the bottom of the screen:

- Discard: the entry is erased and doesn't become part of the patient's chart.
- Back: the healthcare provider returns to the chart to correct the entry.
- Chart New: Changes are saved and a chart for another patient is opened.
- Confirm: Changes are saved and the current patient's chart is continued.

For example, the nurse notices that the significance flag for the patient's weight is not turned on, yet it was noted that the patient lost two pounds in two days, which is probably significant. The nurse can click the Back button and return to the weight entry to turn on the significance flag.

If there were many errors, then selecting Discard and starting over is a better choice. However, if the nurse is satisfied with the information, then he can select Chart New or Confirm. Chart New saves the information and lets the nurse move on to a new patient while Confirm saves the information and returns to the same patient's chart.

8.6.1   Cosigning

Some entries may need to be cosigned by another member of the patient's healthcare team. For example, a nursing assistant is authorized to measure vital signs and enter vital signs into the patient's electronic chart. An RN needs to review and cosign the entry.

Cosigning is performed electronically. With McKesson's charting software, the person cosigning must log into the charting software using his or her own log-in and then display the review screen. Selecting the Cosign button electronically cosigns the entry.

Most charting software prevents an entry that must be cosigned from being saved until the entry is cosigned. The administrator of the charting software assigns personnel authorized to use the charting software into a group based on the person's license and duties. Appropriate rights to features of the charting software are assigned to each group. Before granting access to the charting software feature, the charting software references the group associated with the log-in. These rights are determined by the healthcare facilities policies.

For example, the nursing assistant's log-in is assigned to a group who performs nursing assistant duties and therefore requires access to a specific set of charting software features. One such feature requires entries to be cosigned. Likewise, the RN is assigned to an appropriate group that performs RN duties and has access to a specific set of charting software features that includes access to the Cosign feature.

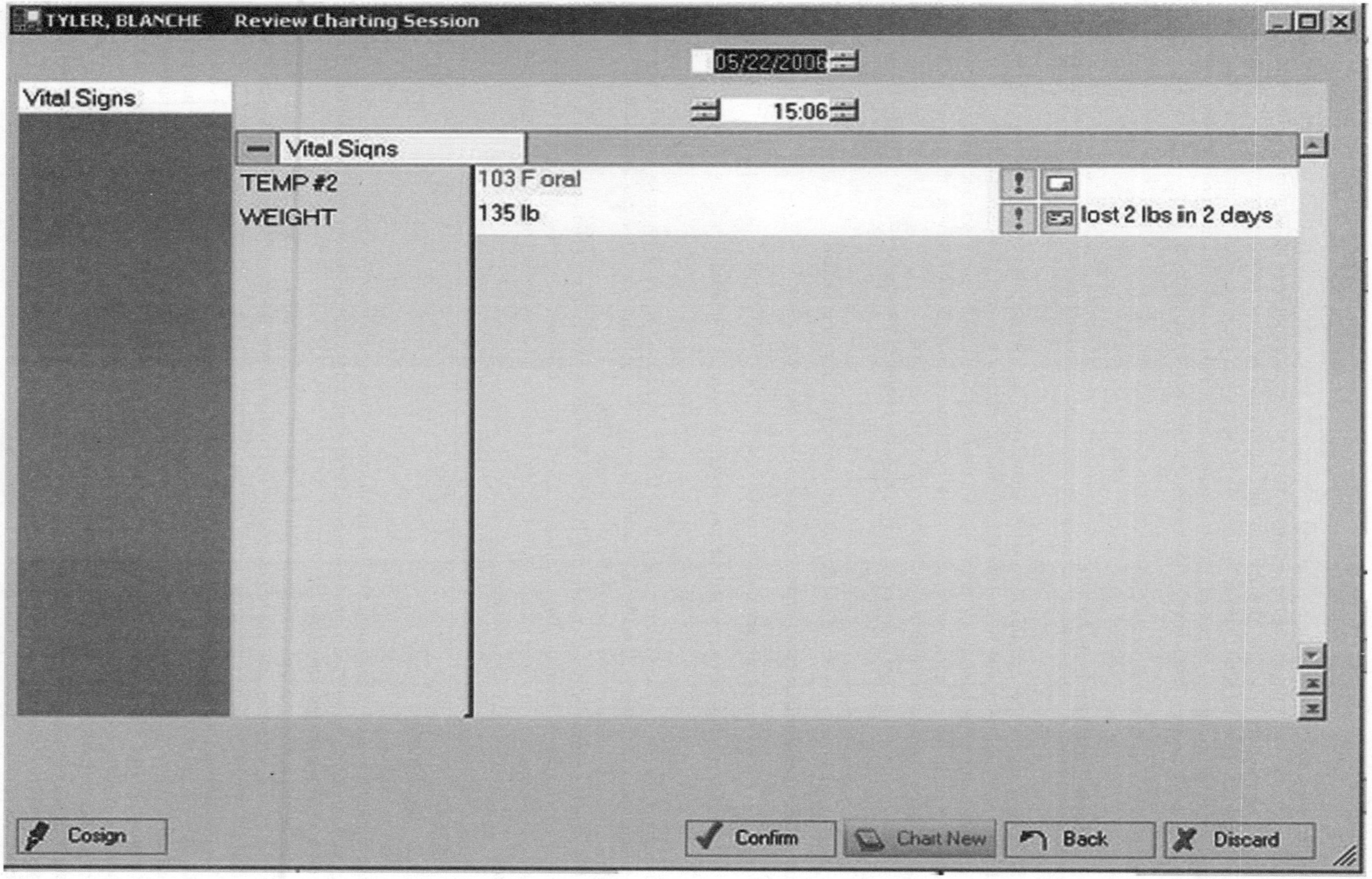
TYLER, BLANCHE Review Charting Session
05/22/2006
Vital Signs
15:06
Vital Signs
TEMP #2
103 F oral
WEIGHT
135 lb
lost 2 lbs in 2 days
Cosign
Confirm
Chart New
Back
Discard
Figure 8.6

8.7   Patient Profile

The patient profile section of the patient's electronic chart is used by clinicians to get a brief overview of the patient before looking at other components of the chart to assess the patient's current status. The patient profile is divided into several tabs of information.

The Patient Detail tab is the initial tab that is reviewed to learn about the patient. This contains the patient's admitting date, admitting complaint, and admitting diagnosis. The admitting complaint is the problem reported by the patient. The admitting diagnosis is the medical diagnosis entered by the practitioner after the patient is assessed. Also listed is the patient's current diagnosis, which may differ from the admitting diagnosis as a result of further testing and assessment.

There are a number of other useful pieces of information on this tab, including the patient's admitting and current weight and height, the patient's medical record number, as well as the patient's unit and attending practitioner.

One of the most important tabs in the patient profile is the Current Allergies tab (Figure 8.7). The Current Allergies tab lists all the patient's allergies as reported by the patient and assessed by the healthcare team. Each allergy appears in a row along with characteristics of the allergy. Characteristics include the type of allergy, the severity of the allergy, and the patient's reaction when exposed to the allergen.

The pharmacy is expected to verify that the patient has an allergy, depending on the healthcare facility's policy. Once verified, the Rx Verified column on the Current Allergies tab is selected. Always assume that the patient is allergic to the allergen even if the Rx Verified column is unchecked.

It is the nurse's responsibility to make sure that newly reported allergies are included in the Current Allergies tab. The nurse does this by selecting the Insert button and then selecting the allergen from the list of common allergens. She then enters characteristics of the allergy. Some allergens are recorded in the system and appears as Coded and others do not.

Allergies that are no longer present can be deactivated by selecting the Active check box in the corresponding allergy row. Only active allergies are displayed by default and appear with a check in the corresponding allergy check box. Removing the check and refreshing the screen enables the nurse to remove the deactivated allergy from the screen.

Active and inactive allergies can be displayed by selecting the allergy history button. Rarely will the nurse need to view inactive allergies; however this feature is useful if the patient reacts to a previously inactive allergen. In this situation, it is possible to recall inactive allergies and then select the Active check box to reactivate the inactive allergy.

The patient's Home Meds tab (Figure 8.8) in the patient profile provides a list of medications that the patient was taking prior to admission to the unit. The Home Meds tab lists meds by name, dose, route, and frequency. In addition, you'll see the date and time of the last time the patient received the dose.

Keep in mind that this list may or may not be inclusive, and information on the list may also be inaccurate. The home medication list is created when the patient is admitted to the facility and based on the best information the nurse has at that time. Ideally, the patient brings a bag of his or her entire collection of home medications and then the nurse enters information on the medication label into the Home Meds tab. The patient then tells the nurse the last time that he or she self-administered the medication.

In reality, the patient may bring in a list of medications or recall names and doses of medication from memory. The admitting nurse needs to assess whether or not the information provided by the patient makes sense. For example, the patient may report taking Baclofen 1000 mg once a day, however Baclofen doesn't come in a 1000 mg dose and is commonly administered three times a day. The nurse does not enter the medication in the Home Meds tab until the medication is verified.

When reviewing the Home Meds tab, the nurse should always verify if the list is complete and accurate by asking the patient to bring in containers of the medication or by getting permission from the patient to contact the patient's pharmacy. The patient's pharmacy is an excellent source for information about the patient's home medication because most patients tend to use the same pharmacy to fill prescriptions even if written by different prescribers.

The nurse is expected to maintain the home medication list during the patient's stay and when the patient is discharged. The patient (or the patient's family) typically identifies additional home medication during the first few days after the patient is admitted to the unit because this information often isn't available during the admitting process.

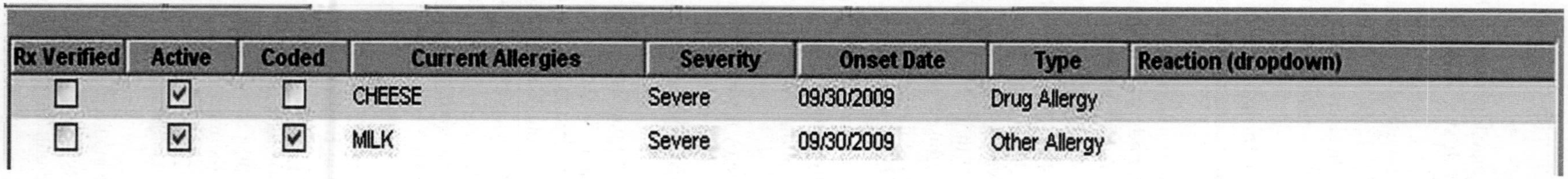

Rx Verified	Active	Coded	Current Allergies	Severity	Onset Date	Type	Reaction (dropdown)
☐	☑	☐	CHEESE	Severe	09/30/2009	Drug Allergy	
☐	☑	☑	MILK	Severe	09/30/2009	Other Allergy	

Figure 8.7

108

Home Meds	Dose	Route	Frequency	Most Recent D
SEROQUEL	300MG	BY MOUTH	BEDTIME	03/20/2011 22:00	Uni
NEURONTIN	300 MG	BY MOUTH	3 XDAY	03/21/2011 13:00	Uni
BACLOFEN	10 MG	BY MOUTH	3 X DAY	03/21/2011 14:30	Uni
LISINOPRIL	10 MG	BY MOUTH	DAILY	03/21/2011 08:00	Uni
VENLAFAXINE	75 MG	BY MOUTH	3 X DAY	03/21/2011 08:00	Uni
NALTREXONE	50 MG	BY MOUTH	DAILY	03/21/2011 11:00	Uni
CARISOPRODOL	350 MG	BY MOUTH	2 X DAY	03/21/2011 15:00	Uni

Figure 8.8

109

The Home Meds tab enables the nurse to change information about the medication such as dose, frequency, or the most recent dose by overwriting the existing information. The nurse can remove the medication from the list by highlighting the medication and selecting the Discontinued button. Likewise, he can enter a new medication by selecting the Insert button.

The Home Meds tab is also used to record a new list of home medications when the patient is discharged from the unit. Upon discharge, the prescriber usually writes prescriptions for medications that the patient will continue at home and instructs the patient to discontinue previous home medication. It is important that the nurse makes these changes in the Home Meds tab before discharging the patient from the unit. When the patient is discharged, the patient's discharge instructions contain the contents of the Home Meds tab. Those instructions along with the prescriptions are given to the patient before the patient leaves the unit.

The patient profile also contains the patient's medical history on the Medical History tab (Figure 8.9). The medical history is divided into systems and disorders. In this illustration, the patient has high cholesterol, hypertension, back pain, and several psychosocial disorders. The patient also had MRSA.

Next to each disorder is a date that the condition was diagnosed based on the patient's recollection. Some patients remember the month and year when they were diagnosed and others remember only the year. The healthcare facility typically has a policy for how to enter the month if the patient is able to remember only the year of the diagnosis. For example, the month will always be January if the actual month is unknown. Dates are sometimes left at zero if the patient is unsure when the disorder was diagnosed.

The Comments column is used to clarify the disorder. The nurse should always enter clarification for each disorder, otherwise the information may be confusing to the healthcare team. Look at Figure 8.9. Does the patient currently have high cholesterol and hypertension? It is impossible to tell because the date is set as zero, and there is no clarification in the comment section. Likewise, there is a history of MRSA but no clarification if the patient completed treatment. Based on the date, it would seem that the patient was treated, but it would be better to have a definitive statement that treatment was completed.

As with the Home Meds tab, the medical history should always be read with skepticism. The information is usually provided by the patient and the patient's family. The diagnosis of the disorder is what they thought the diagnosis was and may not be accurate. The same is true about the date that the diagnosis was reached. Therefore, accept the list as being incomplete. Assume the information is accurate but use critical thinking skills to verify the information.

Next is the Surgeries tab. The Surgeries tab contains a history of surgical procedures performed on the patient usually based on information provided by the patient and family members. Surgeries are listed in the first column followed by the Date and Comment columns, which are very similar to the Medication History tab.

Information on the Surgeries tab poses the same challenges as the Medical History tab in that the information may be incomplete and may need to be verified independently if a medical decision is being based on information in the Surgeries tab.

The last tab is the Immunizations tab. This tab lists all the immunizations that the patient received prior to admissions and during the patient's stay on the unit. There are columns for the names of the immunizations, dates, and comments.

For example, the following would be documented if the TB skin test was administered to the patient:

PPD#1 given in left forearm on 8/1/13 lot# 12344 Exp: 9/14. MYLAN Pharmaceuticals

And then document the reading as:

PPD#1 read on 8/7/13 LFA 0MM induration noted

8.8 Care Plans

A patient presents the practitioner with one or more problems that interferes with the patient's activities of daily living. The practitioner assesses the patient and reaches a diagnosis. A care plan is then developed to treat the patient. A care plan is a roadmap for the healthcare team describing long and short term goals for the patient and interventions that the healthcare team can do to help reach those goals.

Medical History	Date		Comments
Cardiovascular - High Cholesterol	00/00/000	◆	
Cardiovascular - Hypertension	00/00/000	◆	
Musculostoskeletal - Back Problems	05/2007	◆	SLIPPED DISC AND SCIATIA RESULTED FROM AN AUTO ACCIDENT
Musculoskeletal - Falls	00/00/000	◆	HIGH RISK FALL
Psychosocial - Alcoholism	00/00/000	◆	
Psychosocial - Bipolar Disorder	00/00/000	◆	
Psychosocial - Substance Abuse	00/00/000	◆	
Psychosocial - Substance Abuse	00/00/000	◆	H/O ETOH AND OPIATE ABUSE
Infectious Disease - MRSA	02/2005	◆	HOPITALIZED AT SHERMAN OAKS MEDICAL CENTER

Figure 8.9

111

Electronic charting software has a care plan feature that enables the admitting nurse and other members of the healthcare team to enter long and short term goals and corresponding interventions. The initial care plan is created as part of the admissions process. When the patient is assigned to the unit, the patient's name appears on the unit's census and the columns for admissions (AA) and care plan (CP) appear as red squares indicating that the patient still must be admitted to the unit.

Selecting the CP red square causes an empty care plan screen to be displayed. Selecting the Add button enables the healthcare provider to create long- and short-term goals. The initial step is to enter a problem area. Imagine having to sort through a list of medical diagnoses to find the patient's diagnosis. This would be time-consuming. Electronic charting software organizes diagnoses into problem areas by systems or by units of the healthcare facility depending on the desire of the healthcare facility. When the nurse selects the problem area for her unit, the software displays a list of diagnoses common to the unit.

Highlight the diagnosis and press the Select button. The electronic charting software displays corresponding long term and short goals that are typically used for that diagnosis. The nurse is then prompted to enter the rationale for selecting the long and short term goals. The rationale requires the nurse to enter the signs and symptoms and the evidence to support her rationale. The electronic software provides a default rationale, however healthcare facilities usually want to the nurse to tailor the rationale specifically to the patient.

The nurse can select multiple diagnoses from the same screen by highlighting each one and pressing the Select button. Once all the long and short term goals are identified, the nurse selects the Initiate button to create the care plan. The nurse returns to the care plan screen where she will see a list of long and short term goals.

The electronic software will usually enter more long and short term goals in the care plan than is appropriate for a particular patient. The nurse should remove those long and short term goals that don't apply to the patient. This is done by selecting the Inactivate radio button at the bottom of the screen and then selecting the long or short term goal that is to be removed from the care plan. The electronic charting software will place a red X next to the inactive goals.

The next step is to add interventions to each short term goal. This is done by right clicking the short term goal to display a pop-up menu and then selecting Add from the menu to display a list of interventions. Interventions are organized by the titles of the members of the healthcare team. Some interventions are for physicians (MDs) and others for nurses (RNs, RNs/LPNs), social workers (SWs), respiratory therapists (RTs), and others on the team.

Highlight the intervention and press the Select button and the intervention appears under the corresponding short term goal on the care plan (Figure 8.10). It is important to consider which member of the team will perform the intervention before selecting the intervention. For example, there are some interventions that either an RN or LPN can perform. If the selected intervention is an RN intervention then the LPN is excluded from performing this intervention, when in reality it is desirable for either one to be able to perform the intervention.

The care plan is a live document and must be updated during the patient's stay. That is, some long or short term goals are completed before the patient is discharged. Therefore, it is necessary to select the Completed radio button at the bottom of the screen and then select the long or short term goal that is completed. The electronic charting software places a green icon alongside completed long and short term goals.

Likewise, a new long term goal may be added by right clicking the name of the diagnosis on the care plan and selecting Add from the pop-up menu, and then proceeding to select the long term goal and corresponding short term goals from the list as previously described in this chapter. Right clicking the name of a long term goal on the care plan enables the caregiver to follow similar steps to add a corresponding short term goal to the long term goal.

Once the care plan is created, the healthcare team uses the unit's census to document required interventions. The census list has an intervention column (Int) where the color of the square implies the status of the interventions (Figure 8.10). Interventions can be as needed (PRN) or scheduled, depending on the nature of the intervention. For example, the nurse is required to assess the patient's IV site once every shift. This is a scheduled intervention. Alternatively, the nurse is expected to spend at least 15 minutes per shift conversing with the patient as needed. This is an unscheduled or PRN intervention. A green square indicates there are no pending interventions. A yellow square indicates there is a pending intervention. A red square indicates an overdue intervention.

The healthcare team member documents an intervention by double clicking the square in the Int column if the patient's census listing is a list of interventions for the patient. Selecting an intervention displays the intervention on the screen used to document the intervention. These screens are usually part of the Daily Focus Assessment group of tabs that will be discussed in Chapter 9. Document the intervention and then close the screen.

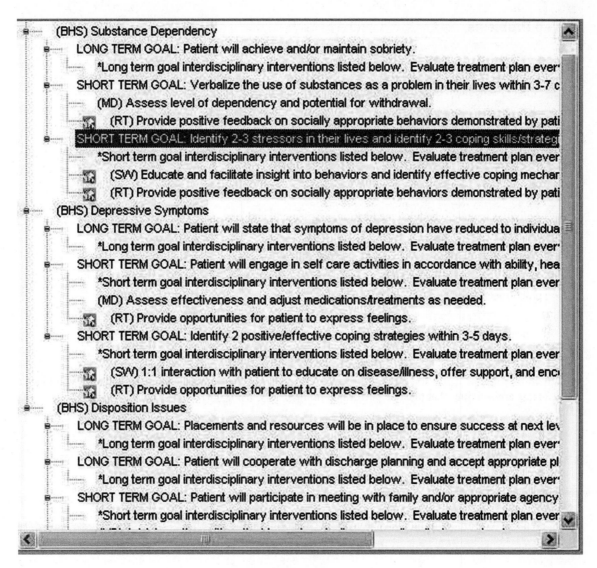

Figure 8.10

The Daily Focus Assessment screen may be displayed by using the toolbar, instead of selecting the Int square and documenting the intervention accordingly; however this approach is discouraged because the results may not show up in a chart audit.

A chart audit is a process where a representative from the healthcare facility or from an outside agency follows the patient's documentation from admission through discharge to examine or track the care the patient received. The auditor assesses how the diagnosis was reached and that the care plan reflects appropriate treatment for the diagnosis. Furthermore, the auditor reviews that corresponding interventions were performed.

Electronic charting software has an auditing feature that assists the auditor examing the electronic documentation. However, interventions are recorded as occurring only if the healthcare team member selects the Int square and corresponding intervention from the intervention list to display the appropriate Daily Focus Assessment screen. If the healthcare team member selects the Daily Focus Assessment from the menu bar, the documentation is not recorded as an intervention and therefore the auditor is led to believe that the intervention was not performed.

When the patient is discharged, the nurse is expected to return to the care plan and mark all the long and short term goals as completed. This is a quick process. The nurse only needs to select the Completed radio button and then click each long term goal. The electronic charting software then marks corresponding short term goals as completed.

Solved Problems

8.1   What is a to-do list?

        A list of scheduled or overdue patient activities that are ordered by the healthcare provider.

8.2   What information is listed on a to-do list?

        The patient's name, unit, room/bed number, medical record number, and a to-do list of pending orders.

8.3   What kinds of activities can be found on a to-do list?

        Activities include scheduled medication, assessment, and labs.

8.4   What information is associated with an Ordered Item?

        The practitioner's order number, enabling the nurse to quickly trace the activity back to the original practitioner's order

8.5   How are rows of patients identified?

        Alternating bands of color making it easy to distinguish patients on the list

8.6   How are activities that must be performed immediately displayed?

        Marked as Stat and highlighted in red

8.7   What is the purpose of the filter bar?

        Used to set criteria for displaying patient information

8.8   What is the purpose of numbers along with categories on the filter bar?

        Indicates the number of items that are in that category

8.9   How is the filter category changed?

        Selecting the appropriate radio button

8.10   What is contained in the Overdues category?

        Activities that are passed their scheduled time.

8.11   What is the purpose of the To Do category?

        Used to display activities that are scheduled or overdue for the current date and time

8.12   What is the purpose of the Changes category?

        Used to display activities that have changed

8.13   What is the purpose of the Activity category?

        Displays all activities that have been scheduled for now and in the future

8.14   What is the purpose of the shift filter?

Displays activities scheduled for the current shift and overdue from previous shifts

8.15   How does the charting software know the date and time of a shift?

The charting software administrator for the healthcare facility defines the shift in the charting software based on the healthcare facility's policy.

8.16   What might be recorded in a log?

An entry is made when the user logs in and logs out. Entries might contain what software is used, what features of the software are used, and what charts are viewed or changed. Nearly everything done electronically may be tracked.

8.17   What is the purpose of the Date and Time range?

This is used to set the "from" and "to" dates and time range to display activities that fall within that range.

8.18   What is the purpose of the Refresh button?

The Refresh button redisplays information on the screen and is used after the filter criteria are reset and whenever the display remains inactive for a period of time. Refresh causes display of recent changes to the patient's chart.

8.19   What is the purpose of Review Mode?

Review Mode is used to display previously entered vital signs and other patient information. The information can be scrolled to view the patient's progress.

8.20   Why are values highlighted in red?

Values highlighted in red are considered significant by the charting software and should be reviewed by members of the healthcare team.

8.21   What is the purpose of the Chart button?

The Chart button is used to enter the Chart Mode where the nurse can enter new information into the patient's chart.

8.22   How would the nurse handle entering vital signs taken at 9 a.m. but entered into the chart at 11 a.m., when the charting software automatically enters the date and time that the entry was made into the chart?

The nurse can correct the date and time by resetting the time of the entry to the time when vital signs were measured.

8.23   How can using a drop-down list save time in entering vital signs and other measurements?

Most frequently selected items on a drop-down list can be set as the default value. The default value always appears at the top of the list in the selection box, eliminating the need to make any selections.

8.24 How would you call attention to an entry?

Selecting the exclamation associated with the entry causes the exclamation to be highlighted in red.

8.25 What occurs when the Save button is selected?

The charting software displays the entered information in a review screen enabling the healthcare provider to discard the entry, return and correct the entry, or save the entry without change and return to the patient's chart or to a new patient's chart.

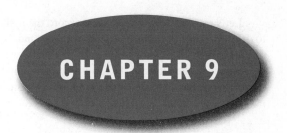

CHAPTER 9

Entering Patient Assessments in Charting Software

9.1   Charting an Assessment

Sections of an electronic chart are similar to tabs in a paper chart. One such section is patient assessment. The section name is based on the charting software. McKesson's charting software calls this section the Assessment and Intervention section.

The section is opened by clicking the section tab. The section is a clinical flow sheet that lists systems in assessment order. McKesson refers to system lists as classes. The clinical flow sheet begins with Neurological and continues in a top-down order corresponding to the order in which a patient is assessed.

Each class opens to a list of specific assessments similar to the vital signs section discussed in Chapter 8 where each class opens a group of vital signs that can be reviewed or a new entry can be made in the chart.

9.2   Entering an Assessment

A list of assessments related to the class that is opened appears on the screen. The actual assessments depend on the charting software and healthcare facility. Charting software manufacturers such as McKesson enable each healthcare facility to customize the list of assessment items.

Select the row containing the assessment to enter a new assessment. This is similar to how the area was displayed on the chart to enter vital signs.

9.2.1   Pick from a List

Charting software removes ambiguities that commonly occur when charting an assessment in a paper chart. The healthcare provider doesn't need to think of the right word to describe the assessment because the charting software has a drop-down list of frequently used assessment results. The list is displayed and then the assessment result is selected.

Selecting the drop-down arrow causes the drop-down list to expand and show all options. These options were added to the list by the charting software manufacturer and by the healthcare facility. This enables finding the proper description for the assessment on the list. If an assessment description is missing from the list, then the nurse can insert a comment into the chart and contact the healthcare facility's administrator of the charting software to ask for additions to the list.

Let's say that the nurse wants to record the patient's level of consciousness. He clicks the Neurological class to display the list of neurological assessments and then clicks the "Neuro assmnt" row to open the assessment area of the chart.

Selecting the arrow in the drop-down list box displays assessment results. If the patient is generally within normal range but there are some exceptions (Figure 9.1), the nurse selects "normal except." The exception is then noted in a comment (see Chapter 8).

9.2.2   Multiple Assessments

A one-word assessment may be adequate to describe an assessment. For example, a patient may exhibit several signs that reflect the patient's level of consciousness (LOC). In such situations a drop-down list of check boxes is used to chart the assessment. Each check box corresponds to an assessment result.

The nurse selects the check box once, and a check appears indicating that the assessment is selected. If the check box is selected again, the check is removed from the check box, indicating that the assessment is no longer selected.

McKesson accommodates multiple assessments by incorporating check boxes in a drop-down list. The healthcare provider selects the drop-down list to display multiple assessments and then selects it again to collapse the drop-down list into a single line on the chart.

9.2.2.1   Picking Multiple Assessments

Here's how an assessment of a patient's level of consciousness is entered. First the nurse selects the LOC line in the Neurological class and then selects the drop-down list. The drop-down list contains a list of assessment results, each as a check box (Figure 9.2).

These include:

- Alert
- Sedated
- Lethargic
- Obtunded
- Restless
- Agitated
- Stuporous
- Combative
- Comatose

Select the appropriate check boxes. If one is selected in error, simply selecting it again removes the check mark. When finished entering the LOC assessment, the nurse selects outside the drop-down list to collapse the drop-down list into a single line on the chart.

9.3   Streamlining Documentation

When the assessment entails multiple assessment results, charting software consolidates multiple results and displays them on the row that contains the assessment making it easy for other members of the healthcare team to quickly review the assessment.

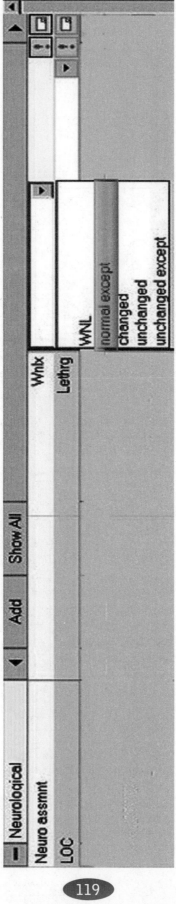

Figure 9.1

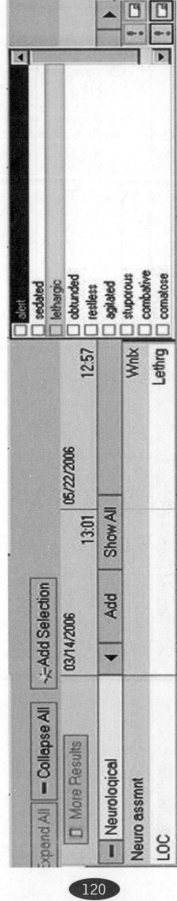

Figure 9.2

Let's say that a patient is gasping and grunting when the sound and breathing portion of the Respiratory assessment is performed. Findings are documented by selecting the sound and breathing row to open its drop-down list. Select "gasping" and then select "grunting." Chart software automatically combines these and displays them on the row (Figure 9.3). Selecting multiple signs and symptoms within a group on the same drop-down list enables the nurse to decrease the time taken to document patient findings.

Another way to streamline the process of charting a patient is to use normal statements. A normal statement is a feature that consolidates typical findings within several categories into one check box item. This enables the healthcare provider to quickly document findings by selecting one item on the electronic chart.

Figure 9.4 illustrates normal statements for a medical surgical unit. Normal statements are divided into systems. A paragraph appears in the normal statement column that describes a normal assessment within the system category. Selecting the normal check box causes the charting software to automatically enter the paragraph into the patient's chart. It isn't necessary to chart further on the patient unless there are abnormal findings. The nurse describes the abnormal findings on the screen that corresponds to the system that he is charting.

There might also be an abnormal status check box that is selected if the patient's condition is not normal. When nurse clicks OK, she'll be brought to the daily assessment screen that contains tabs for each detail assessment, which is where she charts the abnormalities.

Normal statement is a feature that is tailored to the healthcare facility based on the healthcare facility's standard of practice. Some healthcare facilities see normal statements as an efficient tool for documenting normal status of a patient. Other healthcare facilities might see normal statements as a risk because practitioners can use the normal statement as a way to avoid charting a more detailed assessment. For example, the patient's heart rate may be above normal, and other measures are normal. Therefore, it is easy for the practitioner to select normal in the system status column and move on to another chart rather than select abnormal and then enter the detailed assessment.

Likewise, some third party payers may frown upon using normal statements because doubt is raised as to whether or not the practitioner performed the anticipated assessment. Therefore, some healthcare facilities and units within a healthcare facility do not define normal statements.

The healthcare provider will know if a normal statement is defined or not when he opens the assessment feature of the electronic charting software. Depending on the electronic charting software used by the facility, a screen might appear saying there is no normal statement defined and the healthcare provider will be asked to close the screen before proceeding.

9.4 Customize the Assessment

Electronic charting provides a convenient way to choose the assessment screen by presenting available assessments in the form of tabs. Names on the tabs infer assessments available on the tab. At first this may be a little confusing because tab names are shortened and sometimes abbreviated owing to the size of the tab. Once familiar with the assessment screen, the healthcare provider will be able to quickly select the appropriate tab.

Figure 9.5 shows elements of a neurological assessment. In this example, the list of signs and symptoms for most aspects of the neurological assessment is relatively short and therefore displayed as check boxes. The exceptions are describing swallowing, gag reflex, and grip. Each of these requires the selection of signs and symptoms from a drop-down list.

There is a trend among healthcare facilities to directly chart at bedside using electronic charting software. This has two major advantages over paper charting. First, information about the patient is usually made available immediately after saving the assessment. For example, information entered into a tab is saved when moving to another tab. This is beneficial especially in acute and critical care units where multiple medical providers are intervening with the patient simultaneously. Practitioners can access the assessment directly from the computer or have elements of the assessment displayed on a monitor.

The second important advantage of an electronic assessment at bedside rather than paper charting is that the electronic chart displays elements of the assessment. Think of this as a road map guiding the healthcare provider through each assessment. Although some paper charts can also be used as a similar guide, usually paper charting is done at the nursing station and not at bedside. Therefore, the information isn't available during the assessment.

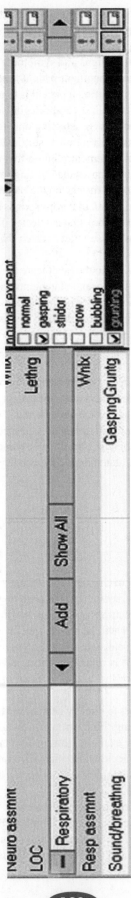

Figure 9.3

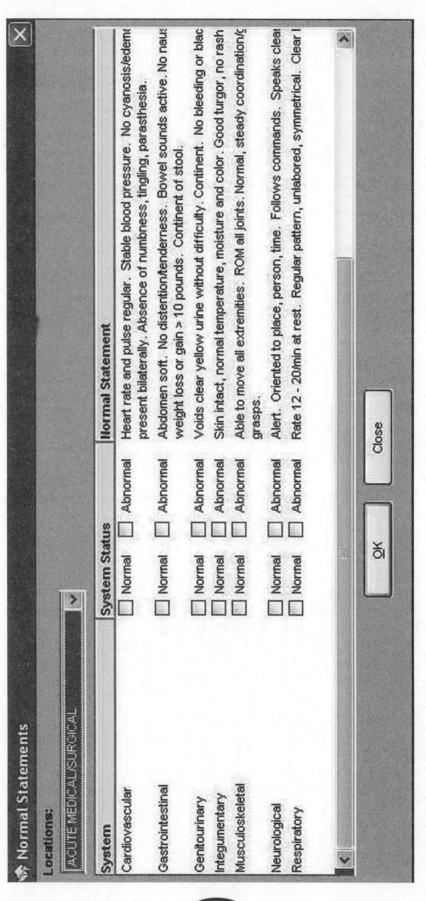

Figure 9.4

123

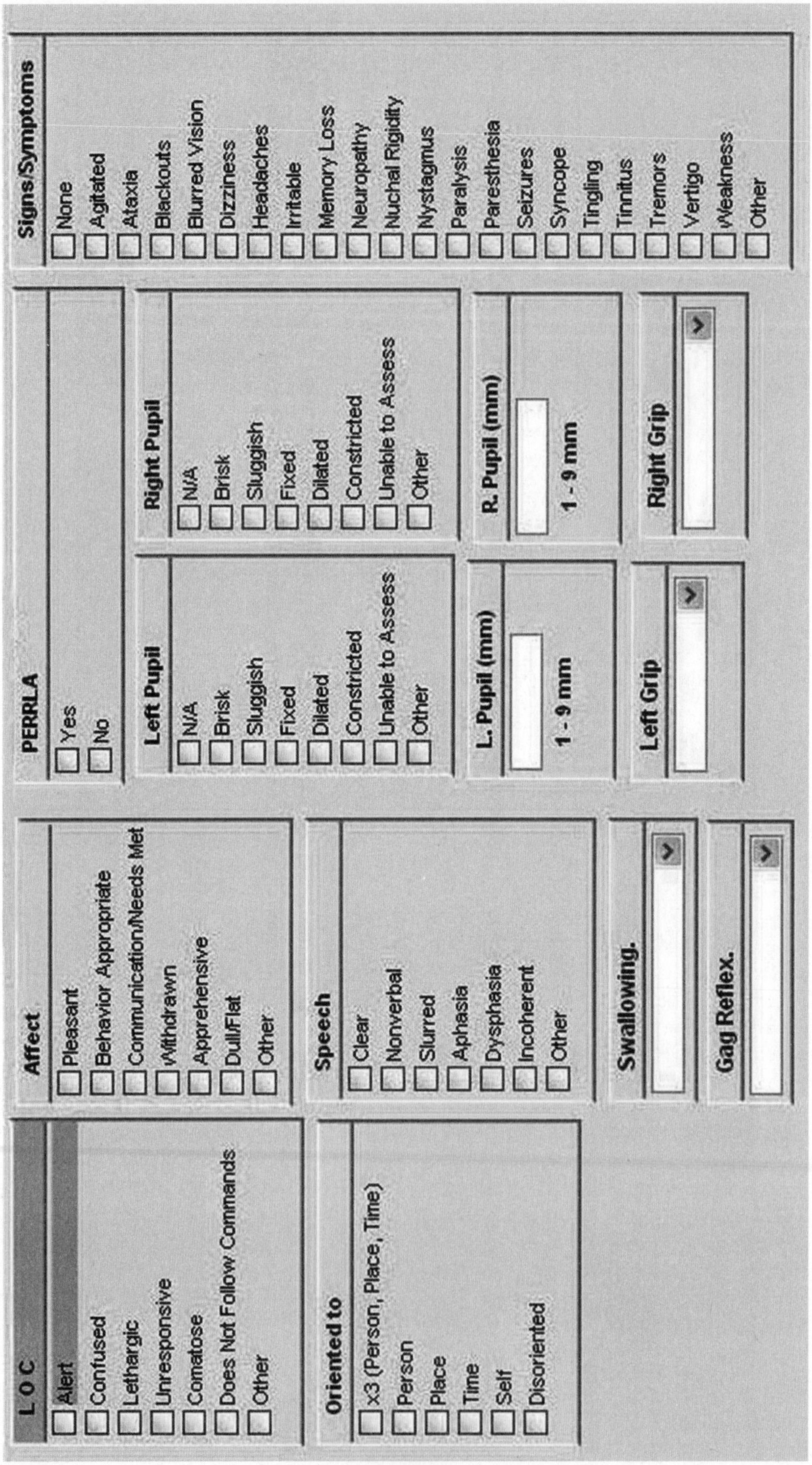

Signs/Symptoms

- None
- Agitated
- Ataxia
- Blackouts
- Blurred Vision
- Dizziness
- Headaches
- Irritable
- Memory Loss
- Neuropathy
- Nuchal Rigidity
- Nystagmus
- Paralysis
- Paresthesia
- Seizures
- Syncope
- Tingling
- Tinnitus
- Tremors
- Vertigo
- Weakness
- Other

PERRLA

- Yes
- No

Right Pupil

- N/A
- Brisk
- Sluggish
- Fixed
- Dilated
- Constricted
- Unable to Assess
- Other

Left Pupil

- N/A
- Brisk
- Sluggish
- Fixed
- Dilated
- Constricted
- Unable to Assess
- Other

R. Pupil (mm)

1 - 9 mm

L. Pupil (mm)

1 - 9 mm

Right Grip

Left Grip

Affect

- Pleasant
- Behavior Appropriate
- Communication/Needs Met
- Withdrawn
- Apprehensive
- Dull/Flat
- Other

Speech

- Clear
- Nonverbal
- Slurred
- Aphasia
- Dysphasia
- Incoherent
- Other

Swallowing.

Gag Reflex.

L O C

- Alert
- Confused
- Lethargic
- Unresponsive
- Comatose
- Does Not Follow Commands
- Other

Oriented to

- x3 (Person, Place, Time)
- Person
- Place
- Time
- Self
- Disoriented

Figure 9.5

124

In the neurological assessment example, the screen is organized into categories of a neurological assessment. These are level of consciousness (LOC), orientation, affect, speech, swallowing, gag reflex, pupil reaction and size, grip, and other signs and symptoms of neurological disorders.

9.4.1 Pressure Ulcers

Patients who are immobile are at risk for pressure ulcers. Electronic charting software helps to identify patients at risk for pressure ulcers by using the electronic version of the Braden Scale. Furthermore, there is an assessment tab that assists in documenting an existing pressure ulcer (Figure 9.6).

The pressure ulcer assessment tab provides a uniform way to document the current status of a pressure ulcer. The wound site is a free-formed text box allowing the nurse to enter a description of the location of the wound. Although the text box is relatively small, up to 255 characters can be entered. Typically nurses will use common abbreviations within the description to make the description concise. Similarly, there is a text box to describe the size of the pressure ulcer. Notice that an example of the format is shown in the title of the text box. This is a recommended format. The electronic charting software will accept any format entered into the text box. The size of the pressure ulcer is noted in centimeters as indicated in the title of the text box. The nurse can enter a value in a different unit, however, if this will be misleading.

The date-acquired element of the assessment can be entered by typing the date or using the scroll arrows to change the date. Typing the date is a more efficient method of entering this information into the electronic chart.

Across the top of the screen are a series of drop-down lists that enable the healthcare provider to select the description of the stage, tissue appearance, depth characteristics, periwound appearance, drainage type, and drainage amount. The advantage of using a drop-down list for these elements of the pressure ulcer is the nurse is ensured of using terms that are commonly used to describe each characteristic of a pressure ulcer. This is an improvement over paper charts that require the writer to remember the commonly used terms as she writes her paper chart assessment. Sometimes the nurse may forget the proper terms that describe the pressure ulcer if she does not assess pressure ulcers frequently in her practice.

Notice the list item in each list of check boxes labeled "Other." The electronic charting software displays the most common assessment term for each element of the assessment based on the practice of that healthcare facility. Electronic charting software, as previously mentioned, can be tailored based on the needs of each healthcare facility. Therefore, the healthcare provider may be familiar with a particular brand of electronic charting software, however the content of screens may differ among healthcare facilities even though each uses the same electronic charting software.

The Other check box enables the healthcare provider to enter his own terms to that element of the assessment. When the Other check box is selected, a text screen appears enabling the healthcare provider to enter his assessment. It is important to realize that the text entered in response to the Other check box will not replace the text "Other."

Each time the pressure ulcer assessment tab is selected, a blank assessment screen will appear. Information from the previous assessment of the pressure ulcer does not appear on the screen. Although some nurses find themselves duplicating information previously entered into the chart, beginning with a blank assessment is beneficial because there is a decrease in charting errors.

A common pitfall of charting an assessment is that some nurses have a tendency to base their current assessment of the patient on a previous assessment. This occurs for a number of reasons that include poor time management resulting in charting at the end of the shift when there is a rush to give reports to the next shift and go home. This is especially true if there has not been any material change from the previous assessment.

Electronic charting software requires the nurse to make her own assessment of the patient and makes it inconvenient to see the previous assessment on the screen. In order to access a previous assessment, the nurse needs to use a reporting feature of the software that displays text of the electronic chart on a different screen and then manually copy the information into the assessment tab.

Also presenting the healthcare provider with a blank assessment tab prevents inaccurate information from a previous assessment from being included in the current assessment. For example if the electronic charting software displayed the previous size of the pressure ulcer, the healthcare provider might inadvertently leave the size unchanged even if the pressure ulcer changed in size.

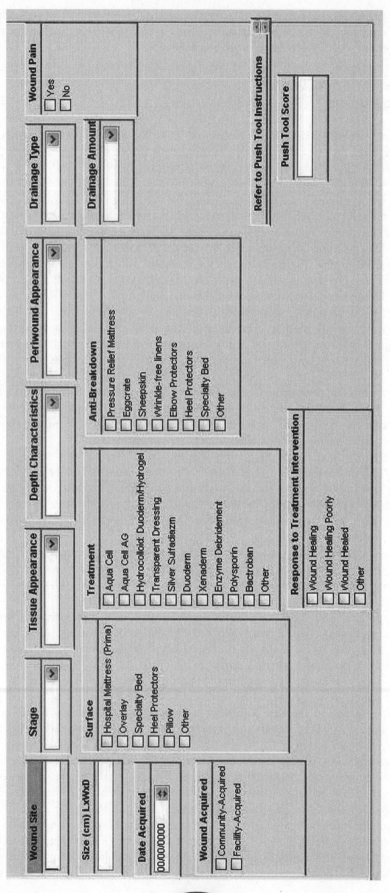

Figure 9.6

9.4.2 Pain Assessment

Pain is the fifth vital sign and is one of the assessments that is most frequently documented in an electronic chart. Typically there are three screens used for pain assessment. Two are used to document pain using either the number pain assessment scale or the FLACC/Wong pain assessment method. The other screen is used to reassess pain within an hour following intervention to relieve the pain.

The pain assessment based on the number scale allows the nurse to document whether or not the patient reported pain and if so the locale and the intensity of the pain described as a value from 1 to 10. In addition, the nurse is asked to record the description of the pain by frequency, character, and precipitating factor. Each of these categories contains check boxes of commonly used terms to describe each category. The nurse is also asked to assess if the patient is oriented to time, place, and person.

A critical element of the pain assessment is pain intervention. In other words, it is necessary to document interventions to reduce the patient's pain. The list of options includes repositioning, medication, rest, diversion, relaxation techniques, heat, cold, or requesting a consultation from a practitioner.

The FLACC/Wong pain assessment tab (Figure 9.7) is used when the patient is unable to fully express pain. You will notice that the FLACC/Wong pain tab has some of the same assessment categories as the pain number tab. In addition, the FLACC/Wong pain tab has categories that describe elements of the FLACC methodology and Wong methodology.

The FLACC/Wong Indicators category describes the status of the patient as disoriented, sedated, asleep, nonverbal, unresponsive, and/or having a language barrier. The Wong-Baker Facial Scale category is used to document the facial scale that is commonly used with children and patients who have difficulty communicating with the practitioner. Although the electronic chart does not have faces for the facial scale, labels of the check boxes correspond to each face in the facial scale.

The FLACC scale section of the tab contains categories that are associated with the FLACC method of pain assessment. Each category reflects an observable behavior that corresponds to the absence of pain or the intensity of pain. Each check box within each category contains a numeric value that when summed creates a FLACC score that corresponds to a pain scale.

The Pain Reassess tab is used to document the outcome of the intervention taken to relieve the patient's pain. All three pain assessment methods are available on this tab. The nurse is asked to select one method, preferably the method originally used to document the pain. The categories are the same as categories on the pain assessment tabs. There is a drawback if you use the Wong-Baker Facial Scale for pain reassessment. The options available are:

- No hurt
- Hurts a little bit
- Hurts a little more
- Hurts even more
- Hurts a whole lot
- Hurts worst

These options are fine for the initial assessment; however on reassessment the patient may not have any change in pain. There is no option that says "hurts the same." This limitation can be overcome by right clicking the category title bar and selecting Group Note from the pop-up menu. The Group Note selection enables free-form text to be entered to describe the pain. A note icon then appears on the category title bar. Selecting the note icon causes the note to be displayed.

9.4.3 Respiratory Assessment

Assessments are made prior to and after treatment, and the treatment itself is documented in an electronic chart. A good example of this practice is with respiratory assessments. Respiratory assessments are performed usually

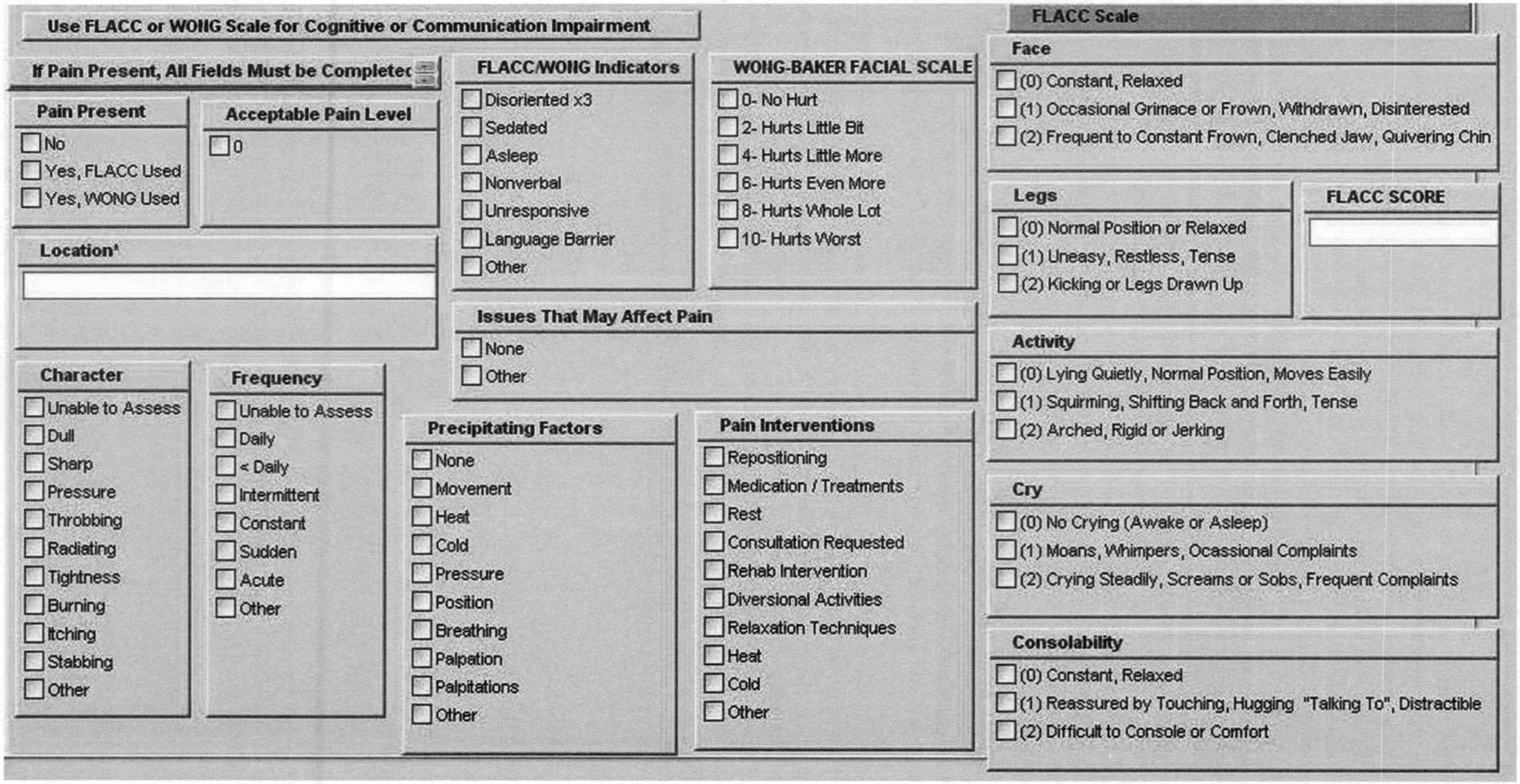

Use FLACC or WONG Scale for Cognitive or Communication Impairment

If Pain Present, All Fields Must be Completed

FLACC Scale

Face
- [ ] (0) Constant, Relaxed
- [ ] (1) Occasional Grimace or Frown, Withdrawn, Disinterested
- [ ] (2) Frequent to Constant Frown, Clenched Jaw, Quivering Chin

FLACC SCORE

Legs
- [ ] (0) Normal Position or Relaxed
- [ ] (1) Uneasy, Restless, Tense
- [ ] (2) Kicking or Legs Drawn Up

Activity
- [ ] (0) Lying Quietly, Normal Position, Moves Easily
- [ ] (1) Squirming, Shifting Back and Forth, Tense
- [ ] (2) Arched, Rigid or Jerking

Cry
- [ ] (0) No Crying (Awake or Asleep)
- [ ] (1) Moans, Whimpers, Ocassional Complaints
- [ ] (2) Crying Steadily, Screams or Sobs, Frequent Complaints

Consolability
- [ ] (0) Constant, Relaxed
- [ ] (1) Reassured by Touching, Hugging "Talking To", Distractible
- [ ] (2) Difficult to Console or Comfort

WONG-BAKER FACIAL SCALE
- [ ] 0- No Hurt
- [ ] 2- Hurts Little Bit
- [ ] 4- Hurts Little More
- [ ] 6- Hurts Even More
- [ ] 8- Hurts Whole Lot
- [ ] 10- Hurts Worst

FLACC/WONG Indicators
- [ ] Disoriented x3
- [ ] Sedated
- [ ] Asleep
- [ ] Nonverbal
- [ ] Unresponsive
- [ ] Language Barrier
- [ ] Other

Issues That May Affect Pain
- [ ] None
- [ ] Other

Pain Interventions
- [ ] Repositioning
- [ ] Medication / Treatments
- [ ] Rest
- [ ] Consultation Requested
- [ ] Rehab Intervention
- [ ] Diversional Activities
- [ ] Relaxation Techniques
- [ ] Heat
- [ ] Cold
- [ ] Other

Precipitating Factors
- [ ] None
- [ ] Movement
- [ ] Heat
- [ ] Cold
- [ ] Pressure
- [ ] Position
- [ ] Breathing
- [ ] Palpation
- [ ] Palpitations
- [ ] Other

Pain Present
- [ ] No
- [ ] Yes, FLACC Used
- [ ] Yes, WONG Used

Acceptable Pain Level
- [ ] 0

Location

Frequency
- [ ] Unable to Assess
- [ ] Daily
- [ ] < Daily
- [ ] Intermittent
- [ ] Constant
- [ ] Sudden
- [ ] Acute
- [ ] Other

Character
- [ ] Unable to Assess
- [ ] Dull
- [ ] Sharp
- [ ] Pressure
- [ ] Throbbing
- [ ] Radiating
- [ ] Tightness
- [ ] Burning
- [ ] Itching
- [ ] Stabbing
- [ ] Other

Figure 9.7

once per shift and as needed for a patient who has a respiratory disorder. Based on the respiratory assessment, the patient will undergo respiratory treatments, although some practitioners will order scheduled respiratory treatments during the acute stages of a respiratory disorder.

Figure 9.8 shows an electronic chart screen that is used to document a respiratory assessment. This assessment can be performed by a practitioner, a nurse, or a respiratory therapist depending on the policy of the healthcare facility. It is essential to indicate whether this is the initial assessment or a subsequent assessment.

If this is the initial assessment, then this assessment will be used by the healthcare team as the baseline assessment for the patient. That is, outcomes of interventions will be measured and compared to the initial assessment to determine if the interventions are resolving the patient's respiratory disorder.

If this is a subsequent assessment, then the results of this assessment will be compared to the initial assessment. Based on the comparison, the practitioner will adjust, continue, or discontinue the prescribed intervention.

Notice that the respiratory assessment focuses both on patients who are on assistance and non-assistance breathing interventions. Patients who are breathing assisted use a supplemental oxygen device and/or a trach tube, if they have had a tracheostomy.

The respiratory assessment requires the healthcare professional to enter the percentage of oxygen and the liters per minute of oxygen that the patient is receiving during the assessment. At times the patient will not receive oxygen during the assessment but will receive oxygen as needed. It is important to accurately document the findings. Therefore, in this situation the nurse enters the percentage and liters per minute of oxygen that the practitioner prescribed as PRN and then right clicks the title bar of the O_2% and O_2 Liters/Min, selects Group Note, and enters a group note indicating that the patient was not receiving oxygen at the time of the assessment but that the patient has been using the prescribed amount of oxygen between assessments. The nurse may also include the time and duration of the oxygen administration. Depending on the policy of the healthcare facility, you will want to perform a respiratory assessment and document accordingly each time oxygen is administered to the patient as a PRN.

For patients who are not receiving respiratory assistance, it is permissible to ignore assessment categories that focus on respiratory assistance. That is, the nurse can simply select Room Air and then enter an assessment in the other respiratory categories.

Remember that many healthcare facilities have adopted a chart-by-exception policy that requires a nurse to elaborate on any abnormal condition that he finds in his assessment. For example, documenting a respiratory assessment that is normal requires checking the following:

- Breath sounds: Clear

- Cough: None

- Secretions: None

- Suction: N/A

- O_2 Device: Room Air

However, the nurse should elaborate if abnormal findings are uncovered. That is, the nurse should select the appropriate check box and then enter a Group Note for the category that further describes her findings. She should be sure to include confirmed and unconfirmed statements the patient makes during the assessment regarding the abnormal finding. The nurse should make sure to place patient comments in quotations in the Group Note and leave her own findings unquoted. This assists other members of the patient's healthcare team in evaluating the assessment.

Only objective statements should be included in the Group Note. Avoid editorializing or summarizing the findings. State facts that expand upon selections made within the category. Save the summary for a progress note.

Respiratory treatments are documented using the Resp Treatment tab (Pt-Resp Treatment). Notice that the respiratory treatment tab contains assessment categories similar to the respiratory assessment tab. In addition, the respiratory treatment tab contains categories related to treatment. These include the type of treatment and the medication administered. Also the indication and rationale for the treatment must be documented.

It is also necessary to document the intervention if treatment was not given. The more common reasons are that the nurse held the treatment or that the treatment was discontinued. If the nurse held treatment, this should be included in a Group Note explaining the rationale for these actions.

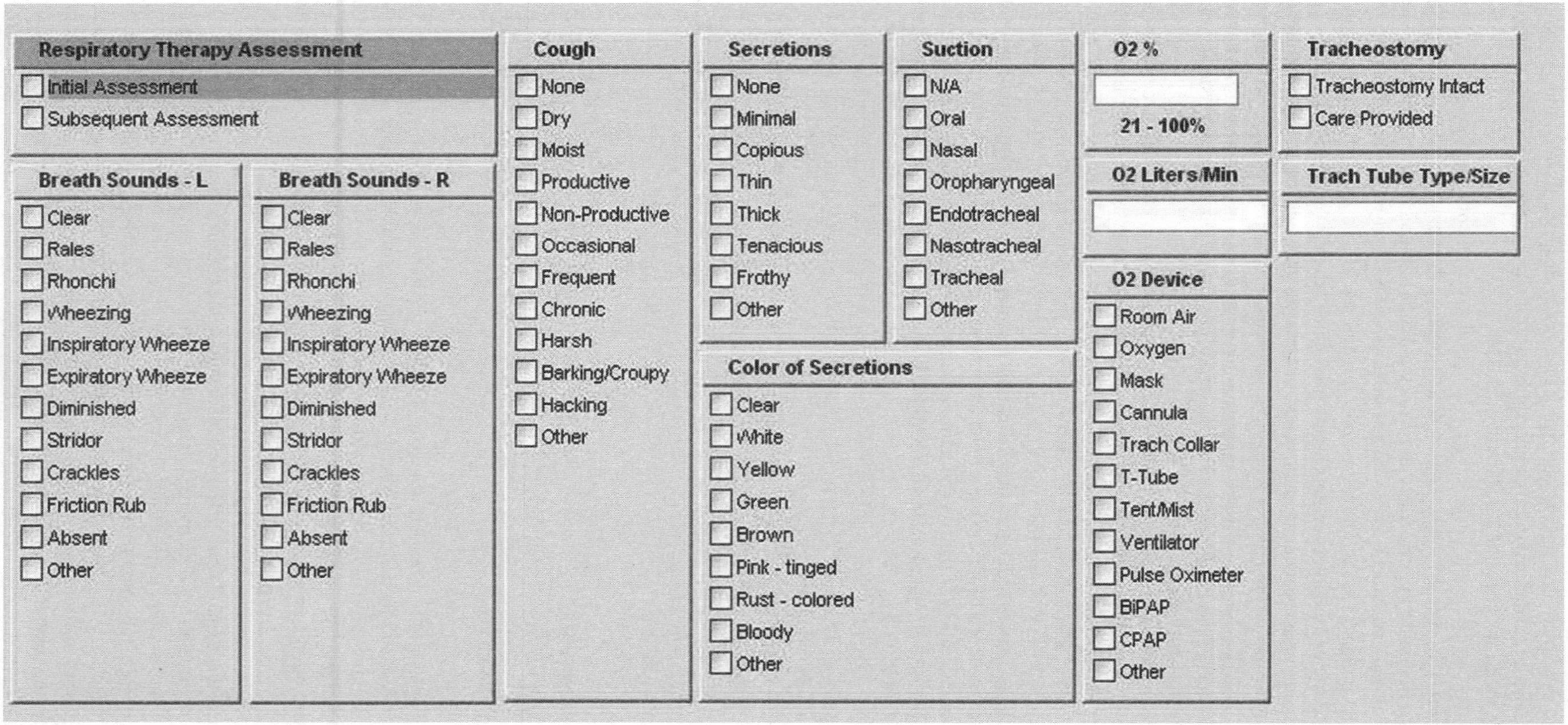

Respiratory Therapy Assessment

☐ Initial Assessment
☐ Subsequent Assessment

Breath Sounds - L

☐ Clear
☐ Rales
☐ Rhonchi
☐ Wheezing
☐ Inspiratory Wheeze
☐ Expiratory Wheeze
☐ Diminished
☐ Stridor
☐ Crackles
☐ Friction Rub
☐ Absent
☐ Other

Breath Sounds - R

☐ Clear
☐ Rales
☐ Rhonchi
☐ Wheezing
☐ Inspiratory Wheeze
☐ Expiratory Wheeze
☐ Diminished
☐ Stridor
☐ Crackles
☐ Friction Rub
☐ Absent
☐ Other

Cough

☐ None
☐ Dry
☐ Moist
☐ Productive
☐ Non-Productive
☐ Occasional
☐ Frequent
☐ Chronic
☐ Harsh
☐ Barking/Croupy
☐ Hacking
☐ Other

Secretions

☐ None
☐ Minimal
☐ Copious
☐ Thin
☐ Thick
☐ Tenacious
☐ Frothy
☐ Other

Color of Secretions

☐ Clear
☐ White
☐ Yellow
☐ Green
☐ Brown
☐ Pink - tinged
☐ Rust - colored
☐ Bloody
☐ Other

Suction

☐ N/A
☐ Oral
☐ Nasal
☐ Oropharyngeal
☐ Endotracheal
☐ Nasotracheal
☐ Tracheal
☐ Other

O2 %

☐ _____
21 - 100%

O2 Liters/Min

☐ _____

O2 Device

☐ Room Air
☐ Oxygen
☐ Mask
☐ Cannula
☐ Trach Collar
☐ T-Tube
☐ Tent/Mist
☐ Ventilator
☐ Pulse Oximeter
☐ BiPAP
☐ CPAP
☐ Other

Tracheostomy

☐ Tracheostomy Intact
☐ Care Provided

Trach Tube Type/Size

☐ _____

Figure 9.8

Any adverse reactions to the medication must also be documented. Common adverse reactions are listed in the electronic chart. Select Other if the reaction is not listed and then enter the reaction as a narrative. Be sure to enter the name of the practitioner and the date and time that the practitioner was notified of the problem.

The final step in documenting the respiratory treatment is recording findings of the patient's breath sounds following treatment. Notice that a slide appears in the right side of the Breath Sounds Post Treatment category box. This indicates that not all responses appear within the category box. Moving the slide down will display other findings that can be selected, the last of which is Other.

9.4.4 Hemodynamic Assessment

Hemodynamics is another field of nursing that focuses on intravenous treatment, blood products, and vascular catheters. There are three screens used to document hemodynamic assessments, each displayed by selecting the appropriate tab from the daily focus assessment screen. Remember that blood products, IV fluids, and fluids administrated through a vascular catheter are fluid intake for the patient and should be recorded on the input/output flow portion of the electronic chart.

These tabs are:

Hemodynamics. The hemodynamics tab focuses on catheter insertion, arterial lines, and central lines. The healthcare provider is expected to document the type and size of catheter and the interventions that he or she performed that involve the catheter. This screen is also used to document outcomes of the intervention.

IV Site. The IV Site tab is used to enter assessments of any IV that has been inserted into the patient. This is where the nurse describes the type and size of the IV and the results of the inspection of the IV site. If there is an infiltrate or phlebitis, the nurse is asked to record the assessment using either the Grade/Infiltration Scale or the Grade/Phlebitis Scale. Grading options for each scale are listed as check box items, making this a relatively straightforward assessment process. Also it is necessary to document interventions taken to resolve any abnormal conditions. Depending on the healthcare facility, the healthcare provider will find a link to standards of practice for IV administration on the IV Site tab. This link enables convenient access to information for administrating an IV. Some healthcare facilities don't offer this link because the linked document is provided by a separate vendor.

Blood Products. The Blood Products tab is used to document when a patient receives a transfusion. This tab is divided into three sections. The first section contains categories that describe the transfusion. The next lists signs and symptoms that the patient may experience. The last section allows the nurse to document interventions taken to resolve adverse signs and symptoms related to the transfusion. Some healthcare facilities require documentation of the transfusion on the transfusion administration record and the transfusion reaction form, both of which are on paper and included in the patient's paper chart.

9.4.5 Diagnostics

Diagnostics consist of procedures and tests whose results will assist the practitioner in determining the patient's diagnosis. The Diagnostics tab is organized into group categories by laboratory procedures, cardiology procedures, respiratory procedures, and radiology procedures. Within each group are lists of tests or procedures in the form of check boxes. The most commonly performed tests and procedures contained in this tab are found here. Obviously these lists are not complete, however the Other option at the end of each list can be selected to document tests and procedures that do not appear within the category. An addition does not appear on the list but instead enables the nurse to write a note that describes the test or procedures. If the nurse wants a new item to appear within the category, he or she can request that the technical staff in the facility add the item to the category.

In addition to these categories, there are the Collected by and Transported categories. The Collected by category lists the title of the staff that collected samples for the test or procedure. The Transported category lists where the sample or patient is going and who or what is involved in the transport.

For example, the patient might be taken to the operating room with the transport and with the cardiac monitor and oxygen. These are items checked off in the Transported category to document the activity.

A common misnomer regarding the Diagnostics tab is that this is used to place the order for a test or procedure. That is, by selecting the EKG check box in the Cardiology Procedures category the EKG technician is notified to come to the patient's bedside and perform an EKG. While this seems logical, the Diagnostics tab is not set up to automatically place the medical order. Likewise by selecting With Transporter in the Transported category, the healthcare provider is not notifying the transportation department to send a transporter for the patient. The Diagnostics tab is strictly used for documenting an event and not ordering an event to occur.

The same activity can be charted on different screens within the electronic medical chart. For example, Pulse Oximeter is listed within the Respiratory Procedures category and also on the vital signs screen. Clinicians would question why it is necessary to select Pulse Oximeter in the diagnostic tab if the value of this reading is documented in the vital signs screen.

One of the goals of electronic charting is to speed the charting process and avoid duplicate charting. However, at times the Diagnostics tab is counter to this objective. Tests and procedures are documented when the medical order is entered elsewhere in the system. The medical order contains the name of the test or procedure. Results of the test or procedure usually contain the name of the person who collected the sample and performed the test or procedure. Therefore, charting on the Diagnostics tab may be considered duplicate charting, which clinicians tend to avoid. A healthcare facility should develop a policy that provides guidance of where the healthcare provider should document an activity.

9.4.6 Treatments

Treatments are documented on the Treatments tab of the Daily Focus Assessment screen. Categories include daily activities, in addition to treatments. For example, there are categories to document bathing and oral and foot care, some of which can be documented as self-care performed by the patient without assistance.

Treatments include care, ostomy care, trach care, pin care, and dressing care. Foley care is documented as to whether or not care was given. Ostomy, trach, and pin care are documented as self-care, partial-care, complete care, or unable-to-give care.

The Dressing Care category contains items that describe the dressing care that was given or describe the state of the dressing. For example, the nurse can document as wet-to-dry dressing, dressing removed, open to air, or topical medication applied. The dressing can be described as dry and intact or dry and sterile.

The Treatments tab is also used to document enema administration and antiembolism care such as applications of Teds to the knee and other antiembolic devices to the patient. There are also categories for Comfort and Range of Motion. The comfort category is used to document the use of a hyperthermia blanket or a hypothermia blanket along with ice pack and soaks. The Range of Motion Performed category is used to record that the patient received active or passive range of motion treatment or refused treatment.

The last category on the Treatments tab is called Treatment Tolerance. This is used to document how well the patient tolerated the treatment. The choices are good, fair, or poor. It is also possible to select Other and enter a free-form description of the patient's response to treatment.

There is also a free-form text box on the Treatments tab that can be used to document care given to the patient that is not identified by a category on the Treatments tab. The text box allows up to 255 characters to describe the treatment.

9.4.7 Cardiac

Documenting the patient's cardiac activity is entered into the Cardio tab of the Daily Focus Assessment (Figure 9.9). The Cardio tab enables a description of the healthcare provider's assessment of the patient's cardiac condition in a number of ways. The first category is called Signs/Symptoms. Although the category title is misleading because other categories also contain signs and symptoms of cardiac disorder, the Signs/Symptoms category lists conditions that might indicate cardiac difficulties.

There are six categories focused on describing the patient's pulse. The first is simply called Pulse. This implies a radial pulse. It is always a good practice to right click the category heading and select Group Note to describe the site of the pulse that was used for this assessment. This enables other clinicians to reassess the findings.

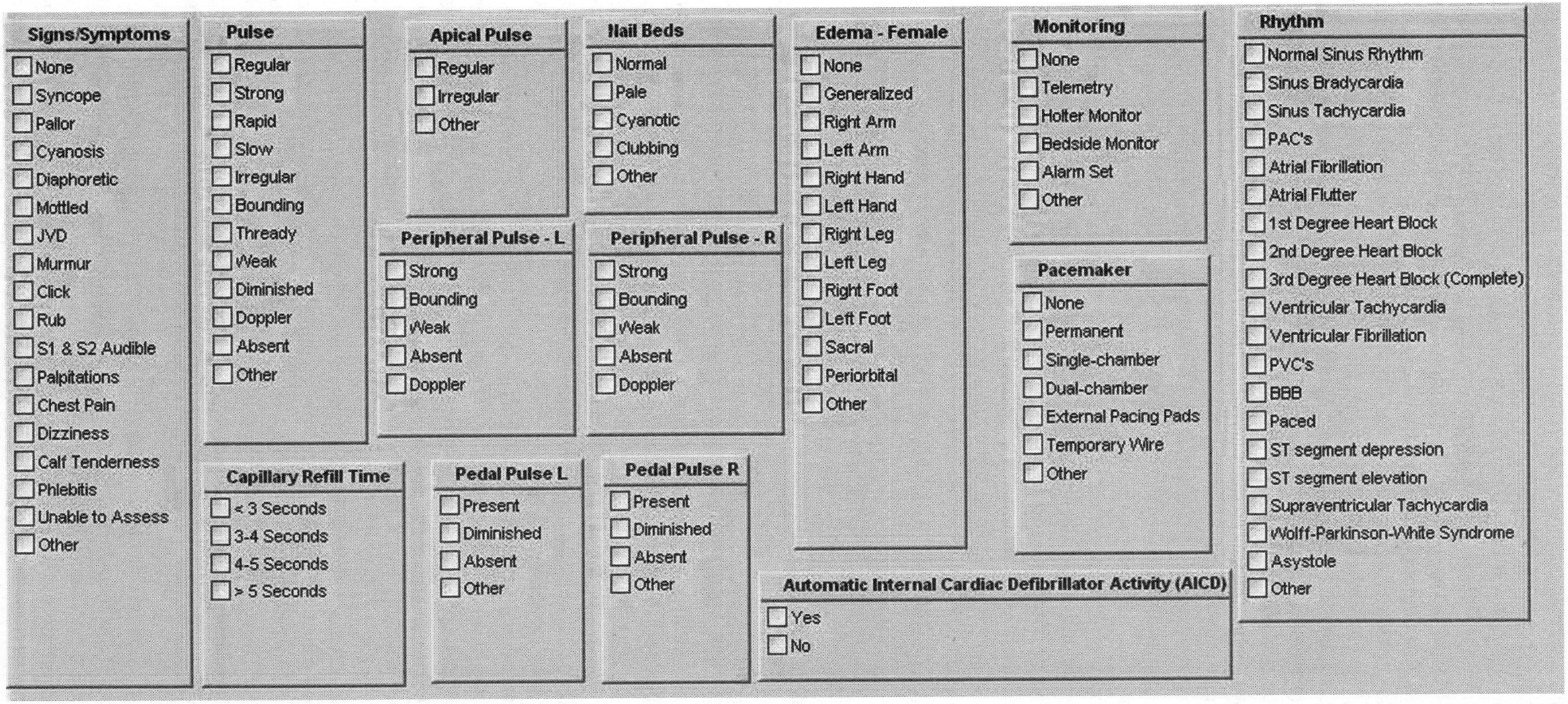

Signs/Symptoms
- [ ] None
- [ ] Syncope
- [ ] Pallor
- [ ] Cyanosis
- [ ] Diaphoretic
- [ ] Mottled
- [ ] JVD
- [ ] Murmur
- [ ] Click
- [ ] Rub
- [ ] S1 & S2 Audible
- [ ] Palpitations
- [ ] Chest Pain
- [ ] Dizziness
- [ ] Calf Tenderness
- [ ] Phlebitis
- [ ] Unable to Assess
- [ ] Other

Pulse
- [ ] Regular
- [ ] Strong
- [ ] Rapid
- [ ] Slow
- [ ] Irregular
- [ ] Bounding
- [ ] Thready
- [ ] Weak
- [ ] Diminished
- [ ] Doppler
- [ ] Absent
- [ ] Other

Capillary Refill Time
- [ ] < 3 Seconds
- [ ] 3-4 Seconds
- [ ] 4-5 Seconds
- [ ] > 5 Seconds

Apical Pulse
- [ ] Regular
- [ ] Irregular
- [ ] Other

Nail Beds
- [ ] Normal
- [ ] Pale
- [ ] Cyanotic
- [ ] Clubbing
- [ ] Other

Peripheral Pulse - L
- [ ] Strong
- [ ] Bounding
- [ ] Weak
- [ ] Absent
- [ ] Doppler

Peripheral Pulse - R
- [ ] Strong
- [ ] Bounding
- [ ] Weak
- [ ] Absent
- [ ] Doppler

Pedal Pulse L
- [ ] Present
- [ ] Diminished
- [ ] Absent
- [ ] Other

Pedal Pulse R
- [ ] Present
- [ ] Diminished
- [ ] Absent
- [ ] Other

Edema - Female
- [ ] None
- [ ] Generalized
- [ ] Right Arm
- [ ] Left Arm
- [ ] Right Hand
- [ ] Left Hand
- [ ] Right Leg
- [ ] Left Leg
- [ ] Right Foot
- [ ] Left Foot
- [ ] Sacral
- [ ] Periorbital
- [ ] Other

Monitoring
- [ ] None
- [ ] Telemetry
- [ ] Holter Monitor
- [ ] Bedside Monitor
- [ ] Alarm Set
- [ ] Other

Pacemaker
- [ ] None
- [ ] Permanent
- [ ] Single-chamber
- [ ] Dual-chamber
- [ ] External Pacing Pads
- [ ] Temporary Wire
- [ ] Other

Automatic Internal Cardiac Defibrillator Activity (AICD)
- [ ] Yes
- [ ] No

Rhythm
- [ ] Normal Sinus Rhythm
- [ ] Sinus Bradycardia
- [ ] Sinus Tachycardia
- [ ] PAC's
- [ ] Atrial Fibrillation
- [ ] Atrial Flutter
- [ ] 1st Degree Heart Block
- [ ] 2nd Degree Heart Block
- [ ] 3rd Degree Heart Block (Complete)
- [ ] Ventricular Tachycardia
- [ ] Ventricular Fibrillation
- [ ] PVC's
- [ ] BBB
- [ ] Paced
- [ ] ST segment depression
- [ ] ST segment elevation
- [ ] Supraventricular Tachycardia
- [ ] Wolff-Parkinson-White Syndrome
- [ ] Asystole
- [ ] Other

Figure 9.9

There are also two categories for peripheral pulse and another two categories for pedal pulse, each focusing on the left or right pulse. The Peripheral Pulse categories have Doppler as an item. Doppler is a check along with a description of the pulse if the pulse was assessed using the Doppler. That is, the healthcare provider needs to check two items if the Doppler is used. Doppler isn't an item in the Pedal Pulse categories, yet sometimes a Doppler is used to assess the pedal pulse if the healthcare provider is able to palpate the pedal pulse. If a Doppler is used for this assessment, it should be stated in a Group Note.

There are also categories used to document Capillary Refill Time and assessment of the Nail Beds. The Edema category contains sites of potential edema. The category name reflects the gender of the patient. This example illustrates a female. The category name will say male for a male patient. The reason for the gender identification is that gender may influence the underlying cause of the edema, and stating the gender reminds the clinician of the gender of the patient.

There are two categories used to document the patient on a cardiac monitor. These are Monitoring and Rhythm. The Monitoring category identifies the type of monitor, if any, that is being used with the patient. The Rhythm category is used to describe the cardiac rhythm as determined by reading the cardiac monitor. It is advisable for the healthcare provider to add a Group Note in the Rhythm category if the patient is on a monitor and is unable to interpret the reading. In the Group Note the nurse simply states that he referred interpretation of the reading to the appropriate clinician. This is an important step because the nurse doesn't want to mislead the reader of the assessment that he placed the patient on a cardiac monitor and then did nothing regarding the reading. The nurse should always document what was done with the reading even if he was unable to interpret the reading himself.

The last set of categories relate to stimulating the patient's heart. These categories are Pacemaker and Automatic Internal Cardiac Defibrillator Activity (AICD). The Pacemaker category describes the pacemaker, if one is used by the patient. The AICD category simple records if an internal cardiac defibrillator is in use by the patient.

9.4.8 Gastrointestinal

The Gastro tab in the Daily Focus Assessment is used to document gastrointestinal interventions and assessments (Figure 9.10). Categories are divided into signs and symptoms, assessment, and treatment. The Signs/Symptoms category focuses on indications of gastrointestinal disorder such as abdominal pain, vomiting, nausea, and constipation. The healthcare provider should be sure to enter a Group Note if she selects a sign/symptom. The Group Note should elaborate the sign or symptom that she selected in the Signs/Symptoms category. It is not sufficient to simply select the sign or symptom without entering a Group Note because the clinician who follows up on the assessment requires details of the findings, more than what can be communicated by selecting a check box item in the category group.

The assessment of the gastrointestinal system is divided into Physical Appearance, Abdomen, Bowel Sounds (one for each quadrant), and Stool Appearance and Consistency. The Physical Appearance category is used to record the stature of the patient such as being overweight or underweight. Items within this category are subjective because it is not necessary to specify the patient's weight, height, or the patient's Body Mass Index (BMI), which are recorded in the Vital Signs screen. Therefore, it is important to follow the healthcare facility's policy regarding how to objectively define a patient as being overweight or underweight or normal weight.

The Bowel Sounds categories provide four options: normal sounds, hyperactive sounds, hypoactive sounds, and absent of bowel sounds. Each category focuses on upper/lower, left/right quadrants of the abdomen.

The Stool Appearance category and the Consistency category are used to describe the patient's stool. Stool Appearance is defined by color and whether or not mucus is present. Consistency is defined by the form and if the stool is bloody or not. Depending on the clinical environment, a patient is sometimes hesitant and embarrassed to ask the nurse to view his or her stool. It is important that the nurse sees the stool before documenting the stool appearance and consistency. The patient's statement should not be accepted as fact. Clinicians require objective evidence in order to follow up with further assessments and treatment. If a patient reported an unusual bowel movement, the nurse should document the patient's claim in the Stool Appearance and Consistency categories; however a Group Note should be included that states this was not witnessed. This approach records the event yet tells the clinician that the event was not verified. The clinician then can determine the proper follow-up assessment and treatment. The Gastro tab also provides a category to record the date of the patient's last bowel movement.

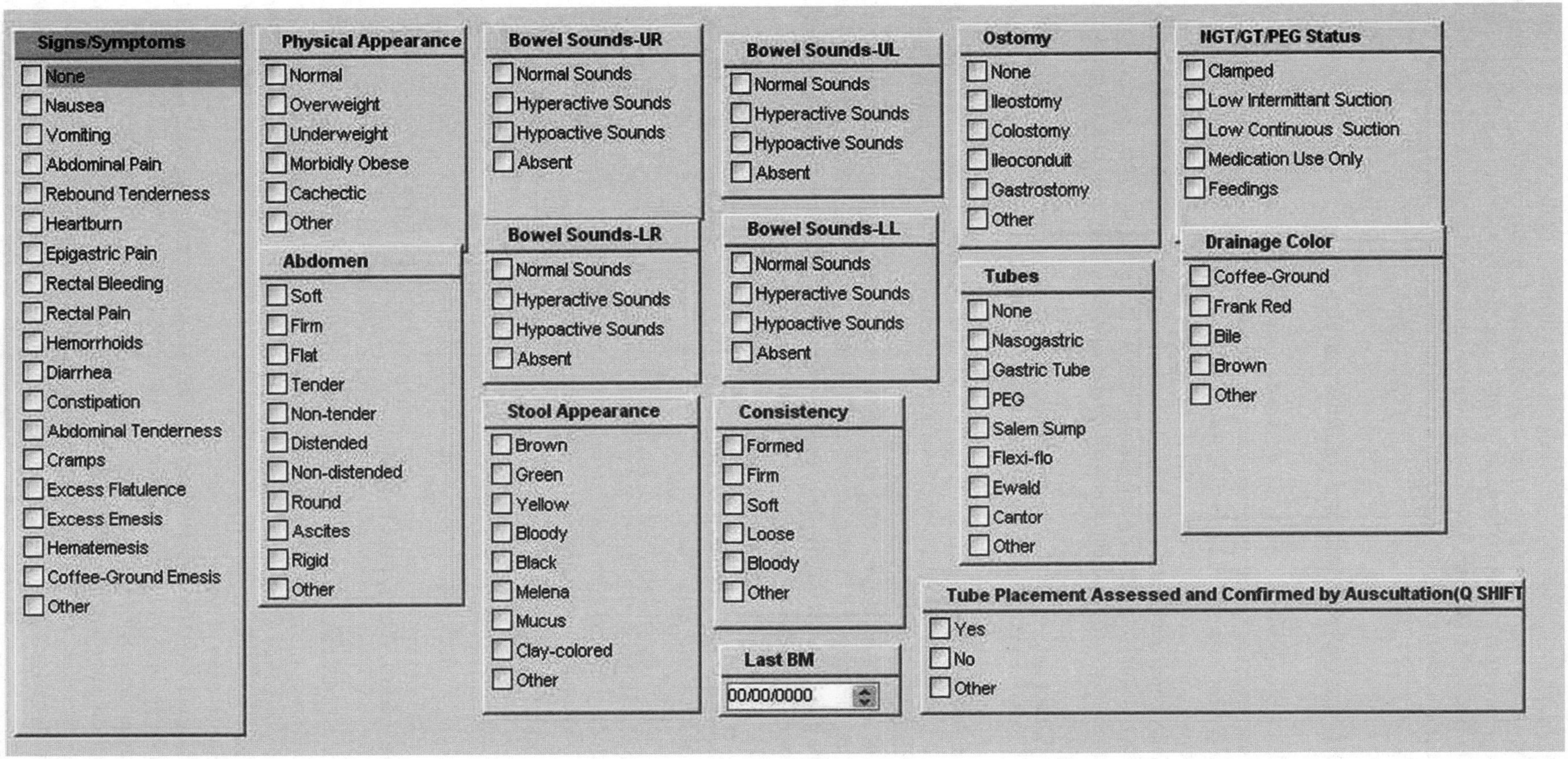

Signs/Symptoms
- [ ] None
- [ ] Nausea
- [ ] Vomiting
- [ ] Abdominal Pain
- [ ] Rebound Tenderness
- [ ] Heartburn
- [ ] Epigastric Pain
- [ ] Rectal Bleeding
- [ ] Rectal Pain
- [ ] Hemorrhoids
- [ ] Diarrhea
- [ ] Constipation
- [ ] Abdominal Tenderness
- [ ] Cramps
- [ ] Excess Flatulence
- [ ] Excess Emesis
- [ ] Hematemesis
- [ ] Coffee-Ground Emesis
- [ ] Other

Physical Appearance
- [ ] Normal
- [ ] Overweight
- [ ] Underweight
- [ ] Morbidly Obese
- [ ] Cachectic
- [ ] Other

Abdomen
- [ ] Soft
- [ ] Firm
- [ ] Flat
- [ ] Tender
- [ ] Non-tender
- [ ] Distended
- [ ] Non-distended
- [ ] Round
- [ ] Ascites
- [ ] Rigid
- [ ] Other

Bowel Sounds-UR
- [ ] Normal Sounds
- [ ] Hyperactive Sounds
- [ ] Hypoactive Sounds
- [ ] Absent

Bowel Sounds-LR
- [ ] Normal Sounds
- [ ] Hyperactive Sounds
- [ ] Hypoactive Sounds
- [ ] Absent

Bowel Sounds-UL
- [ ] Normal Sounds
- [ ] Hyperactive Sounds
- [ ] Hypoactive Sounds
- [ ] Absent

Bowel Sounds-LL
- [ ] Normal Sounds
- [ ] Hyperactive Sounds
- [ ] Hypoactive Sounds
- [ ] Absent

Stool Appearance
- [ ] Brown
- [ ] Green
- [ ] Yellow
- [ ] Bloody
- [ ] Black
- [ ] Melena
- [ ] Mucus
- [ ] Clay-colored
- [ ] Other

Consistency
- [ ] Formed
- [ ] Firm
- [ ] Soft
- [ ] Loose
- [ ] Bloody
- [ ] Other

Last BM
00/00/0000

Ostomy
- [ ] None
- [ ] Ileostomy
- [ ] Colostomy
- [ ] Ileoconduit
- [ ] Gastrostomy
- [ ] Other

Tubes
- [ ] None
- [ ] Nasogastric
- [ ] Gastric Tube
- [ ] PEG
- [ ] Salem Sump
- [ ] Flexi-flo
- [ ] Ewald
- [ ] Cantor
- [ ] Other

NGT/GT/PEG Status
- [ ] Clamped
- [ ] Low Intermittant Suction
- [ ] Low Continuous Suction
- [ ] Medication Use Only
- [ ] Feedings

Drainage Color
- [ ] Coffee-Ground
- [ ] Frank Red
- [ ] Bile
- [ ] Brown
- [ ] Other

Tube Placement Assessed and Confirmed by Auscultation(Q SHIFT
- [ ] Yes
- [ ] No
- [ ] Other

Figure 9.10

The remaining category groups focus on assistive devices inserted into the patient. These include various types of ostomy, tubes, status, and a description of drainage from these devices. For the ostomy and tubes, the nurse selects the type, if any, that is present. The status category is used to record the status of gastric tubes, nasogastric tubes, and PEG tubes. The Drainage Color category provides selections of coffee-ground, frank red, bile, and brown. The nurse can also record tube placement assessments in the Gastro tab.

9.4.9   GIGU (Gastrointestinal and genitourinary)

The Genito tab is where the nurse documents signs and symptoms of urinary disorder, urinary tubes and drains, and female discharges. The Signs/Symptoms category lists common indications of urinary problems that are reported by the patient or identified by the clinician.

Three category groups focus on urinary status. These are Urinary Elimination, Urine Appearance, and Urine Color. The Urinary Elimination category is where the nurse documents if the patient is continent or incontinent and has a Foley catheter, ostomy, or is undergoing hemodialysis. Urine appearance is recorded as clear, cloudy, bloody, or unable to obtain if the patient has not urinated for the assessment. Urine color contains a list of common colors of urine.

The Tubes/Drains category is used to identify the type of tube or drain used by the patient to urinate. This category is not used to record the assessment of the tube or drain. It is simply used to document if one is in use by the patient.

Notice that the Foley catheter and ostomy can be documented on several tabs in the Daily Focus Assessment. It is important that the healthcare facility or unit set policy as to which tab to use when documenting these devices, otherwise there will be no continuity in documentation.

The Female Discharge category is the place where the nurse documents if the patient has a vaginal discharge or urethral discharge or if menses are present. The nurse should be sure to describe the discharge in detail in a Group Note if she selects an item in this category, because the clinician will require more information about the discharge than simply that the discharge is present.

9.4.10   Muscles and Skeletal

The Musculoskeletal tab is used to report on the patient's muscles and skeletal assessments. Similar to the other tabs, the muscles and skeletal assessment begins with the Signs/Symptoms category of muscular and skeletal disorders that lists common indicators of problems with muscles and bones.

Also on this tab are categories to document mobility, movement, and strength of arms and legs. Each is recorded separately. The last category on the tab focuses on ambulatory aids. This is where the nurse documents if the patient uses a wheelchair, cane, walker, or other devices that enable the patient to be more mobile.

9.4.11   Eyes, Ears, Nose, and Throat

Assessments of the eyes, ears, nose, and throat are entered into the EENT tab on the Daily Focus Assessment. There are several categories on the tab for each assessment. The eye assessment enables the nurse to report on eye pain and discharges and whether or not the patient wears glasses or has any common eye disorder. The nurse can also note the visual acuity of the left and right eyes. In addition, he can record any drainage from the eye in the Eye Drainage category.

The ear assessment also focuses on common problems such as pain, discharge, and hearing loss. There is also an Ear Drainage category used to describe any substance that is excreted from the ear. The description is reported by amount and color.

The Throat category is used to describe the patient's throat. The throat is reported as redness, white patches, hoarseness, pain, and if there is an exudate discovered. The EENT tab is also used to document nasal and sinus discharges, gum, teeth, and tongue assessments in addition to the condition of the patient's mucosa.

9.4.12   Lesions and Body Markings

When a patient is admitted to a unit, it is important to document any lesions and body marking, such as tattoos and scars, for two important reasons. First, the lesion or body marking may interfere with treatment or indicate prior treatment that the patient has not mentioned during the admission process. For example, it is not unusual for a patient to forget to mention an appendectomy that occurred a decade or more ago. Assessing the patient's body would reveal scars from the surgery.

The second reason for documenting lesions and body markings during the admissions assessment is to record the status of the patient when admitted. Any new lesions or body markings documented on discharge likely occurred during the patient's stay in the healthcare facility. Lesions and body markings at discharge that were not reported on admission must be explained in the chart. For example, a tattoo may be used to help identify the target site in radiation therapy. The tattoo is a body marking that is placed on the patient during the stay. In some situations, the patient may have fallen during his or her stay, resulting in injuries that left a scar.

Lesions and body markings are documented using the Lesions tab (Figure 9.11). The Lesions tab displays anatomically correct images of the body. In this example, the images are of a male patient. There is an anterior and posterior image.

Move the cursor over the image and the cursor changes to a crosshair. Position the center of the crosshair over the area of the body that contains the lesion or body marking and right click the mouse to display a list of descriptions. The list of descriptions contains common types of lesions and body markings. Select the appropriate description and the electronic charting software places an abbreviation for the description at the site of the crosshair. If the appropriate description is not found on the list, the nurse selects Other to enter a description. This process is repeated to document other lesions and body markings. If there are no lesions or body markings, then the nurse selects the No Lesions Noted check box.

A good practice is to explain the lesions in a Group Note so that the clinician has a more thorough understanding of the lesion or marking.

9.4.13   Bedside Procedures

The Bedside Procedures tab is where the nurse documents commonly performed medical activities for the patient. These procedures are not activities of daily living. Instead, they are the insertion of an NG tube or a Foley catheter and more involved procedures such as paracentesis, dialysis, and lumbar puncture.

The first category of this tab is called Bedside Procedures and contains a list of procedures that are frequently performed at bedside. This is used to record that the procedure took place. The nurse will need to add a Group Note to further explain the rationale for the procedure and provide other information about the procedure. The Procedure Tolerance category can be used to indicate how well the patient tolerated the procedure.

The NG Tube Insertion category lists types of NG tubes enabling the nurse to select the NG tube type that was inserted into the patient. The Tube Placement Assessed and Confirmed by Auscultation category records that the healthcare provider confirmed placement of the NG tube. There is a Drainage category that contains descriptions of common drainage from the NG tube. The drainage recorded here is the initial drainage. Additional drainage is documented in the appropriate systems tab.

The Foley Catheter Insertion category has a similar list except this contains types of Foley catheters. Two other categories related to this are Urine Color and Urine Appearance. These are used to document urine returned from the initial insertion. Subsequent urine is documented in the Genito tab.

The last category on this tab is Procedure Performed By. This contains a list of clinicians by title that can perform some or all of these bedside procedures. Traditionally the nurse documents by title and not the name of the clinician. If the healthcare facility requires the nurse to document the name of the clinician, then this is done in a Group Note.

9.4.14   Behavioral Assessment

Electronic charting is used in psychiatry to document the patient's status and any interventions that might occur to assist the patient in regaining calm and controlled behavior. The BIRP1 tab is one of the components of the electronic chart used to record the behavioral assessment (Figure 9.12).

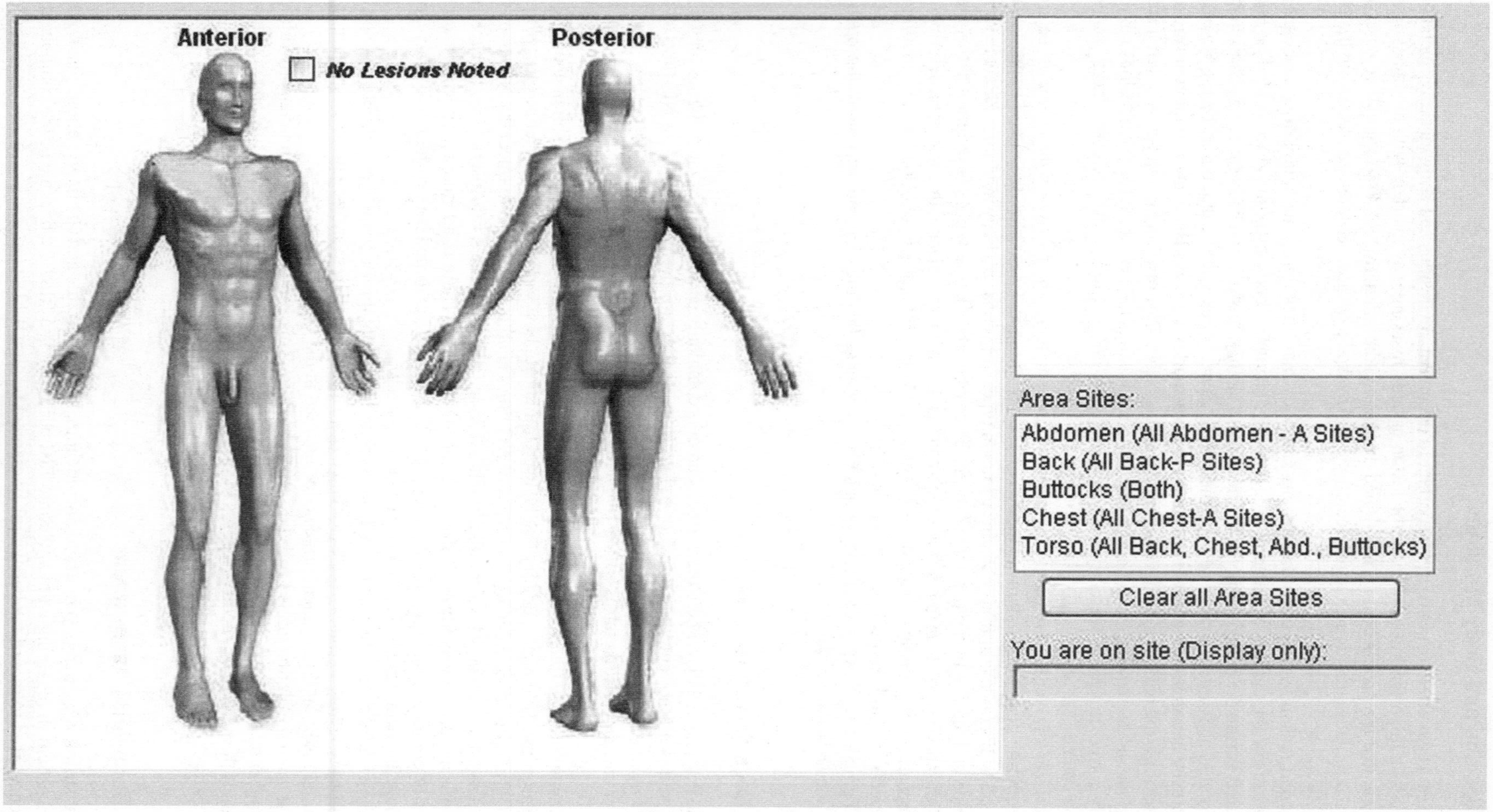

Anterior ☐ *No Lesions Noted*

Posterior

Area Sites:

Abdomen (All Abdomen - A Sites)
Back (All Back-P Sites)
Buttocks (Both)
Chest (All Chest-A Sites)
Torso (All Back, Chest, Abd., Buttocks)

Clear all Area Sites

You are on site (Display only):

Figure 9.11

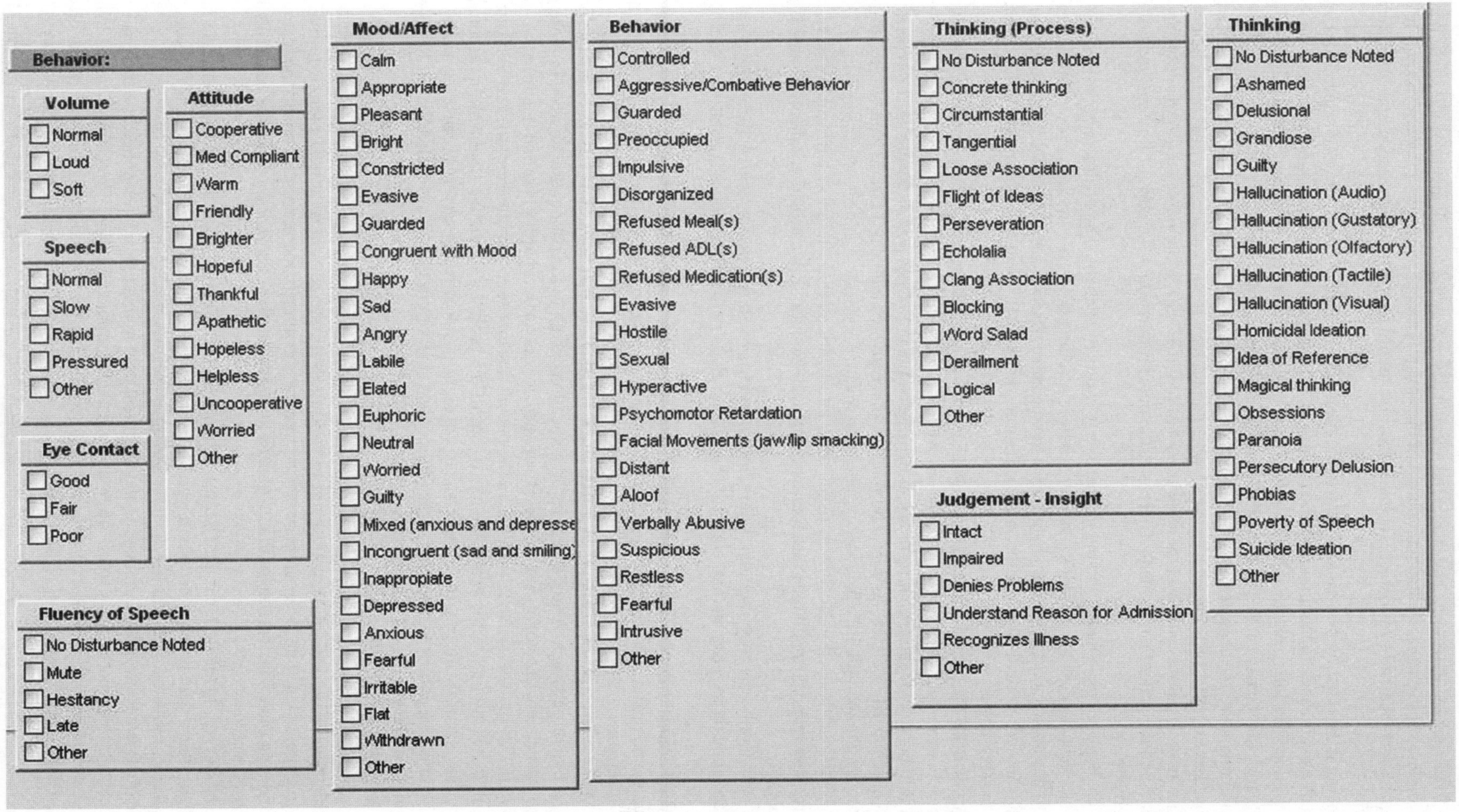

Behavior:

Volume
- [ ] Normal
- [ ] Loud
- [ ] Soft

Attitude
- [ ] Cooperative
- [ ] Med Compliant
- [ ] Warm
- [ ] Friendly
- [ ] Brighter
- [ ] Hopeful
- [ ] Thankful
- [ ] Apathetic
- [ ] Hopeless
- [ ] Helpless
- [ ] Uncooperative
- [ ] Worried
- [ ] Other

Speech
- [ ] Normal
- [ ] Slow
- [ ] Rapid
- [ ] Pressured
- [ ] Other

Eye Contact
- [ ] Good
- [ ] Fair
- [ ] Poor

Fluency of Speech
- [ ] No Disturbance Noted
- [ ] Mute
- [ ] Hesitancy
- [ ] Late
- [ ] Other

Mood/Affect
- [ ] Calm
- [ ] Appropriate
- [ ] Pleasant
- [ ] Bright
- [ ] Constricted
- [ ] Evasive
- [ ] Guarded
- [ ] Congruent with Mood
- [ ] Happy
- [ ] Sad
- [ ] Angry
- [ ] Labile
- [ ] Elated
- [ ] Euphoric
- [ ] Neutral
- [ ] Worried
- [ ] Guilty
- [ ] Mixed (anxious and depressed)
- [ ] Incongruent (sad and smiling)
- [ ] Inappropiate
- [ ] Depressed
- [ ] Anxious
- [ ] Fearful
- [ ] Irritable
- [ ] Flat
- [ ] Withdrawn
- [ ] Other

Behavior
- [ ] Controlled
- [ ] Aggressive/Combative Behavior
- [ ] Guarded
- [ ] Preoccupied
- [ ] Impulsive
- [ ] Disorganized
- [ ] Refused Meal(s)
- [ ] Refused ADL(s)
- [ ] Refused Medication(s)
- [ ] Evasive
- [ ] Hostile
- [ ] Sexual
- [ ] Hyperactive
- [ ] Psychomotor Retardation
- [ ] Facial Movements (jaw/lip smacking)
- [ ] Distant
- [ ] Aloof
- [ ] Verbally Abusive
- [ ] Suspicious
- [ ] Restless
- [ ] Fearful
- [ ] Intrusive
- [ ] Other

Thinking (Process)
- [ ] No Disturbance Noted
- [ ] Concrete thinking
- [ ] Circumstantial
- [ ] Tangential
- [ ] Loose Association
- [ ] Flight of Ideas
- [ ] Perseveration
- [ ] Echolalia
- [ ] Clang Association
- [ ] Blocking
- [ ] Word Salad
- [ ] Derailment
- [ ] Logical
- [ ] Other

Judgement - Insight
- [ ] Intact
- [ ] Impaired
- [ ] Denies Problems
- [ ] Understand Reason for Admission
- [ ] Recognizes Illness
- [ ] Other

Thinking
- [ ] No Disturbance Noted
- [ ] Ashamed
- [ ] Delusional
- [ ] Grandiose
- [ ] Guilty
- [ ] Hallucination (Audio)
- [ ] Hallucination (Gustatory)
- [ ] Hallucination (Olfactory)
- [ ] Hallucination (Tactile)
- [ ] Hallucination (Visual)
- [ ] Homicidal Ideation
- [ ] Idea of Reference
- [ ] Magical thinking
- [ ] Obsessions
- [ ] Paranoia
- [ ] Persecutory Delusion
- [ ] Phobias
- [ ] Poverty of Speech
- [ ] Suicide Ideation
- [ ] Other

Figure 9.12

The BIRP1 tab has categories that enable the nurse in describing the overall mental status of the patient during assessment. These categories include volume of the patient's voice, pattern and fluency of speech, and how well the patient maintained eye contact. The nurse can also record the patient's attitude, mood, and affect as well as behavior.

Thinking is assessed by process such as tangential thinking, flight of ideas, or word salad. Thinking is also recorded as a disturbance in the thinking process such as various types of hallucination, paranoia, phobias, and suicide ideation. The Judgment-Insight category is used to summarize the assessment of the patient's judgment and whether or not the patient has insight into his or her own mental disorder.

It is important that the documentation focus on the clinical judgment during the period that the nurse assessed the patient. For example, on admission to the unit the patient may report audio and visual hallucinations, paranoia, and suicide ideations. However, none of these are reported during the nurse's assessment because of the effectiveness of the patient's treatment. Therefore, the nurse reports only the current findings and not findings of a different period.

The challenge of psychiatric nursing is to properly assess the patient. The healthcare provider must assess the patient's behavior and the patient's statements before reaching his or her findings. For example, the patient may report that audio hallucinations no longer exist yet the nurse observes the patient holding a conversation with someone who does not exist. When the nurse questions the patient about this observation, the patient might admit to hearing voices.

It is critical that the nurse includes a Group Note for any abnormal document that provides a narrative for the assessment. For example, selecting Hallucination (Audio) is not sufficient documentation that the patient hears voices. It is important to report whether or not those were command voices and if so were those voices telling the patient to hurt himself or others. As a general rule, the nurse always includes a Group Note if selecting an item in the category does not tell the whole story of the assessment.

The BIRP2 tab is used to document psychiatric interventions that the nurse performed for the patient. Psychiatric interventions are divided into four categories: Behavioral, Educational, Medication, and Treatment Plan Review.

The Behavioral category includes interventions such as safety checks, active listening, food, group therapy, and thought assessment, and corrective actions such as redirection, boundary settings, setting limits, and time-outs.

The Educational category focuses on educational topics such as disease process, illness management, stress management, and medication education. This category is also used to document providing emotional and family support.

The Medication categories are used to record any medical issues that the patient reported and who was contacted regarding those issues. Also PRN and stat medications given to the patient are recorded in these groups. Scheduled medications are not document here since they are not an exception to normal treatment.

There are two categories used to document the patient's response to the intervention. The first category in this area of the electronic chart is where the nurse records the patient's subjective statement in response to the treatment. The patient's statement is an important aspect of the psychiatric assessment because the statement provides insight into the patient's thought process. The second category in this area is called Patient Response and lists common responses that patients have to these interventions.

The last categories address the patient's treatment plan. Once a patient has a diagnosis, the treatment team formulates a plan for treating the patient, which is called a treatment plan. After an intervention, the nurse and the treatment team decide whether or not to continue with the current treatment plan or to modify the patient's treatment plan. The Plan category is used to enter the nurse's recommendations to the team regarding the treatment plan. The Treatment Plan Changes category is where the nurse enters the actual changes to the plan.

The last category in that group is the Treatment Plan Review category. Depending on the healthcare facility's policy, the treatment plan is reviewed once a week in acute units and monthly in subacute units. This category is used to document what occurred during the treatment plan review.

Some treatment teams find documenting the treatment plan in this tab redundant because there is a section of the electronic chart that focuses solely on treatment plans and interventions. The compromise is that documenting treatment plan reviews and changes are performed using the treatment plan section of the electronic chart. The Daily Focus Assessment is used to document interventions required by the treatment plan.

9.4.15 Progress Notes

Another way to document the patient assessment is to use a progress note. A progress note is a free-form text editor that enables the healthcare provider to enter a narrative about the patient. There are various thoughts about using a progress note for documentation. Some nurses believe that a progress note provides a summary of the patient assessment and is easy to access and read. That is, the progress note tells the whole story about the patient's status. This is similar to writing the patient assessment in a progress note in a paper chart. From this point of view, to simply "click" the assessment is providing a lesser quality assessment.

Other nurses find that writing a progress note for each patient is time consuming and is useful only if something exceptional has occurred with the patient. The Daily Focus Assessment provides a more efficient and effective way to document. Selecting items from a list of common assessments conveys the same information as writing a progression note, especially if Group Notes are used to further explain abnormal findings.

Progress notes are troublesome. Patient and facility statistics cannot be generated if documentation is in a progress note because computers have a difficult time searching for keywords and organizing data if the data is stored in free-form text. For example, the medical team may want to know if a specific treatment is successful. A report can be created that creates an aggregated timeline of assessments for patients who receive the treatment and if the patients improved according to the assessments. This could not be done for assessments that were recorded as progress notes because the information needed for the report is not segregated and uniform. Uniformity is another benefit of selecting items within an assessment category list. Each clinician uses the same sets of words when describing his or her assessment of the patient compared with no standardization of words used in a progress note.

Depending on the electronic charting software, assessments appear in reports as a list of selected items from the assessment category or in a computer-generated narrative. In either case, the clinician reading the report is able to understand the status of the patient.

Therefore, the best approach to use is to select items from the assessment category list and include a Group Note to explain any abnormalities related to assessments within that category. In addition, progress notes may be used to explain situations that related to abnormalities across assessment screens. That is, the progress note is used to summarize a complex assessment. However, the nurse should also document the assessment in the appropriate tab and category. The progress note is a supplement to, not an alternative to, assessment tabs and categories.

9.5 Something Unusual

The nurse can elaborate an assessment by inserting a comment. As illustrated in Chapter 8, a comment can be up to 255 characters and directly associated with each item on the chart.

In McKesson's software, the nurse selects the rightmost icon in the row to open the comment text box and then begins typing the comment. She selects elsewhere on the chart to resume charting. Selecting the comment icon again allows the nurse to see and modify the comment.

If the assessment result is unusual, the urgent flag is set to alert other members of the healthcare team. The exclamation mark icon in McKesson's charting software is the urgent flag. Selecting the exclamation mark icon sets the urgent flag on, and selecting it again turns off the urgent flag.

9.6 Saving and Reviewing

When the nurse is finished entering his assessment results in the chart, he selects Save at the bottom of the chart to display the Review screen. The Review screen is similar to the review screen illustrated in Chapter 8 (Figure 8.6).

The nurse can select:

- **Discard**: the entry is erased and doesn't become part of the patient's chart.
- **Back**: the healthcare provider is able to return to the chart to correct the entry.
- **Chart New**: Changes are saved and the nurse begins to chart a new patient.
- **Confirm**: Changes are saved and the nurse continues to chart the current patient.

Solved Problems

9.1   What is a section of an electronic chart?

A section is similar to sections of a paper chart that are identified by tabs.

9.2   How is a section of an electronic chart opened?

The section tab is usually selected by clicking the tab.

9.3   How is a section structured?

A section is structured in a clinical flow sheet that lists systems in the order of assessment.

9.4   What does McKesson call a system list?

A system list is called a class.

9.5   What approach is taken by a clinical flow sheet?

The clinical flow sheet begins with Neurological and continues in a top-down order corresponding to the order in which a patient is assessed.

9.6   What is displayed when a class is selected?

A list of assessments specific to the class is displayed.

9.7   Who determines the list of assessments that appear in the electronic chart?

The software manufacturer and the healthcare facility determine this list.

9.8   How is a new assessment entered?

A new assessment is entered by selecting the row containing the assessment.

9.9   How does charting software remove ambiguities common in paper charting?

Charting software uses drop-down lists of frequently used assessment results.

9.10   Who determines the assessment results that appear in the drop-down lists?

The software manufacturer and the healthcare facility determine these lists.

9.11   Is it possible to insert an assessment result to a drop-down list?

Not directly; however it is possible to request that the software administrator insert the assessment result to the drop-down list.

9.12   How is a drop-down list expanded?

Selecting the drop-down list, usually by clicking it, causes the drop-down list to expand.

9.13   What are two formats used in a drop-down list?

A list enabling one selection and a drop-down list enabling multiple selections that are usually in the form of check boxes are two formats.

9.14   How does the healthcare provider remove an assessment result recorded in the form of a check box if the selection was made in error?

Selecting the check box a second time removes the check mark.

9.15   How is a drop-down list closed?

Selecting the drop-list again collapses the drop-down list into a single line on the chart.

9.16   How does charting software display multiple assessment results?

Multiple assessment results are automatically consolidated on the assessment row.

9.17   How would the nurse call attention to an abnormal assessment?

Selecting the exclamation mark associated with the assessment causes the exclamation mark to be highlighted in red.

9.18   How would the nurse reverse an alert signal in the chart regarding an assessment result?

Selecting the exclamation mark a second time will return the exclamation mark to its normal color.

9.19   How would the nurse record an assessment if the assessment result does not appear on a drop-down list?

The assessment result would be recorded as a comment.

9.20   How is a comment entered into the chart?

The rightmost icon in the row is selected to open the comment text box, and then the nurse begins typing the comment. Selecting elsewhere on the chart resumes charting. Selecting the comment icon again allows the nurse to see and modify the comment.

9.21   What is the limitation of entering a comment into the chart?

The comment must be less than 255 characters.

9.22   What would the healthcare provider do if he realized he entered the assessment in the wrong patient's chart?

The nurse would select the Discard option in the review screen.

9.23   What would the nurse do if she realized she entered an error in the assessment of the correct patient's chart?

The nurse would select Back from the review screen.

9.24   What is the best way to prevent errors from entering the chart?

Careful review of all entries in the review screen before confirming the entry is the best way to prevent errors.

9.25   What would the nurse do if after reviewing his entries he realized he forgot to enter an assessment for the patient?

The nurse would select Confirm from the review screen. This saves the current entries and returns the nurse to the patient's chart to continue charting.

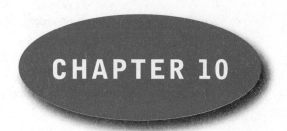

CHAPTER 10

Entering Medication Administration in Charting Software

10.1 Definition

Miscommunication among the practitioner, the medication order, the pharmacist, and the nurse who administers the medication can lead to medication errors. Charting software reduces the opportunity for medication errors by providing a clear channel for communication among the healthcare team and by applying built-in controls to automatically enforce the five rights of medication administration.

10.2 Enforcing Rights of Medication Administration

The five rights of medication administration guarantee that

- The right medication is administered
- To the right patient
- At the right time
- In the right dose
- Using the right route

Charting software automates medication by:

- Using bar codes to identify the patient
- Using bar codes to identify the medication

- Verifying against the medication order:
  ○ The patient
  ○ The medication, dose, and route
  ○ The date and time to administer the medication
  ○ The current date and time

10.2.1　Identify the Patient

In many facilities information that identifies the patients is printed on the patient's wristband and encoded into a bar code. The nurse must verify the identity of the patient typically by asking the patient's name and date of birth and comparing that information to the wristband. Information on the wristband may not be correct.

Once the patient is identified manually according to the facility's policies, then the bar code on the patient's wristband is scanned. A handheld bar code reader that is attached to the computer is placed over the patient's wristband (Figure 10.1). Pressing the button on the bar code reader causes a red light to shine on the wristband, which reads the bar code and beeps when it is finished reading it.

10.2.2　Identify the Medication

Once the bar code on the patient's wristband is scanned into the computer, the charting software displays the patient's electronic medical record listing medications that are due to be administered enabling the nurse to gather the medication.

The medication label identifies the medication and dose. The packaging of the medication implies the route. The medication label also has a bar code (Figure 10.2) that identifies the medication and dose.

Select a medication that is due to be administered and scan the bar code on the medication label similar to how the bar code on the patient's wristband is scanned.

10.2.3　Comparing the Patient and Medication

The charting software retrieves the medication order written by the practitioner, and medication information entered by the pharmacist.

Inside the computer, a number of things happen.

The current date and time are compared to the date and time that medication is scheduled to be administered. This assures that the medication is being administered at the proper time.

The medication is compared to medications that were already administered to the patient. This determines if the patient already received the scheduled medication and thereby prevents the patient from receiving a second dose.

The medication, dose, and route are compared to the medication order written by the practitioner to determine if the medication that is at bedside conforms to the medication order.

The medication is compared to other medications that the patient was recently administered to identify contraindications. For example, the medication may have to be given at least an hour after another medication was administered to the patient. The charting software will detect if an hour has passed.

A warning message is displayed on the computer if the charting software detects that any of the five rights of medication administration is being violated. If no violations occur, then the charting software automatically displays that the medication was administered to the patient.

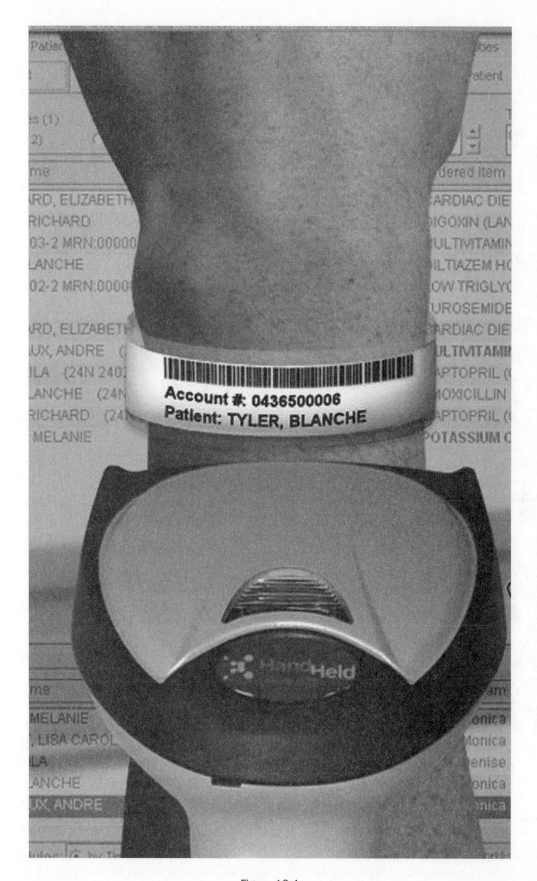

Figure 10.1

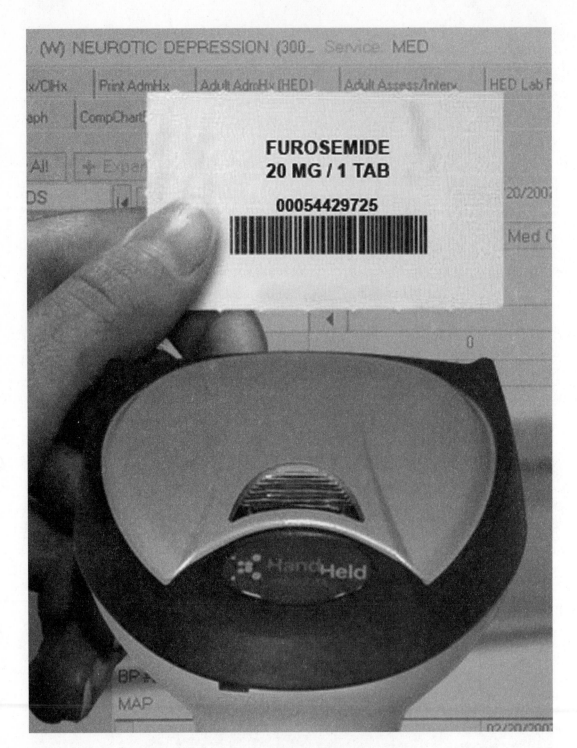

Figure 10.2

10.3 Medication Administration Workflow

Charting software is not a substitute for following standard medication administration procedures. The workflow for medication administration is the same regardless if there is a paper medication administration record or an electronic medication administration record.

Begin the workflow by reviewing the medication order. The medication order appears on the patient's electronic chart and is entered into the charting software either by the practitioner or by the nurse under the practitioner's direction.

Once the medication order is reviewed, collect the medication from the medication room in the unit. Depending on the nature of the medication, the route used, and how the medication is provided by the pharmacy, the nurse may have to prepare the medication in the medication room.

Take the medication to the bedside and verify the right patient, the right medication, the right dose, the right time, and the right route.

Scan the patient's bar code into the charting software, which displays the patient's chart. Compare information displayed on the patient's chart with the information on the patient's wristband to make sure that the right patient is being addressed.

Scan the bar code on the medication label into the charting software. The charting software opens areas on the chart where the nurse can enter information about how the medication was administered. Some charting software may require that the medication bar code be scanned twice as a check and balance to assure that the medication is correct for the patient per the medication order.

Administer the medication to the patient. Charting software gives a place to enter comments alongside the medication in the chart such as how well the patient accepted the medication.

The nurse selects the Confirm button on the charting software indicating that he is finished administering medication to the patient. The charting software saves the medication administration record to the patient's chart. Once saved, this information is available to members of the patient's healthcare team from computers on the hospital's computer network.

10.4   Documenting Medication Administration

The following is a walk through the process using McKesson's charting software. Althoug healthcare facilities may use different charting software, most are likely to work similar to McKesson's charting software.

Blanche Tyler is the patient. It is 7:50 a.m. Ms. Tyler is to receive a furosemide 20-mg tablet at 8 a.m. The status is Scheduled indicating that she has not yet received the medication.

The nurse gets the medication from the medication room. No medication preparation is required since this is a tablet. The nurse returns to the patient's bedside and scans the patient's wristband bar code into the charting software. The charting software displays Ms. Tyler's medication orders (Figure 10.3).

Scanning the bar code on the furosemide label causes a medication administration entry to open in Ms. Tyler's chart. By default, the charting software displays the name of the medication, the dose, and the route to be used. In this example, the medication ordered is 20 mg per tablet to be administered orally.

The nurse can overwrite the dose and number of tablets because the pharmacy might have delivered a different dose per tablet (Figure 10.4). For example, the pharmacy might have delivered 10 mg per tablet. The patient is to receive two tablets of 10-mg tablets rather than one 20-mg tablet. This complies with the medication order; however, the nurse must overwrite the default values displayed by the charting software to reflect medication that was administered to the patient.

In the upper-right corner of Figure 10.4 is an envelope icon, which when selected displays a notepad where a comment may be entered. A comment reflects something unusual that occurred when trying to administer this medication to the patient, such as the patient's refusal to take the medication.

An exclamation mark appears to the left of the comment icon. This is selected if the nurse wants to call the comment to the attention of other members of the healthcare team. The nurse should always notify the practitioner personally whenever a problem arises when administering medication to the patient. She should not simply enter a comment and set the exclamation mark.

The number and types of fields that are available to document the medication administration varies depending on the nature of the medication and the medication order. For example, the nurse won't see a field for pump setting unless the medication is being administered by IV.

The nurse scans the medication's bar code again, and the charting software displays a preview of information that will be recorded in the patient's chart. This reflects any changes that were made to the entry in the previous screen. The nurse doesn't do anything with this screen.

Patient Name	Scheduled	Group	Status	Ordered Item	Dose/Duration	Route	Prty Freq (Rate)	Order #'s
TYLER, BLANCHE	02/21 08:00	MEDS	Scheduled	FUROSEMIDE	20 MG=1 TAB	ORAL	RTN BIDBL	7734 (4)
24N 2402-2 MRN:000001064	02/21 10:00	MEDS	Scheduled	DILTIAZEM HCL (CARDIZEM SR)	90 MG=1 CP12	ORAL	RTN Q12H	7733 (3)
	02/21 12:00	DTY	Scheduled	LOW TRIGLYCERIDE			DTY TIMED MEALS	2359966
		MEDS	Scheduled	FUROSEMIDE	20 MG=1 TAB	ORAL	RTN BIDBL	7734 (4)
	02/21 14:00	MEDS	Scheduled	AMOXICILLIN (AMOXIL)	500 MG=1 CAP	ORAL	RTN Q8H	7716 (1)
	----------	MEDS	PRN	ACETAMINOPHEN	650 MG=(2 x 325 MG TA	ORAL	PRN Q6HP	7732 (2)

Figure 10.3

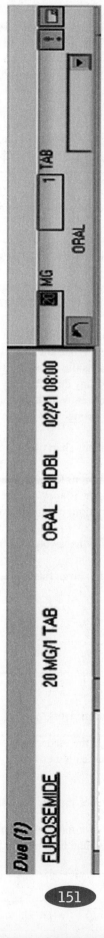

Figure 10.4

151

Now it is time for the nurse to administer the furosemide to Ms. Tyler. After administering the medication, she selects the Confirm button on the bottom of the screen (Figure 10.5) to save the information.

If something noteworthy occurs such as Ms. Tyler refusing to take the medication, then the nurse can select the Back button to return to the previous screen where she can enter a comment and change other information associated with administering medication to Ms. Tyler. If the nurse does this, she will need to scan the medication bar code once she is finished changing the information in the charting software.

10.5   Recovering when Problems Occur

Failures can occur when using charting software, however charting software manufacturers provide built-in workarounds to recover from a failure.

A common failure with charting software is when the bar code reader is unable to read the patient's bar code on the wristband. The wristband may have been damaged, which is common when a patient has a long stay in a healthcare facility.

Failures reading bar codes on medication labels are rare because medication packages are less likely to be exposed to the environment for long periods of time because medications are typically replenished to the unit twice a day.

There are two ways to notice when the bar code reader fails to read the patient's bar code. First, there is no audible beep when scanning the bar code. The beep signals that the bar code has been successfully read. No beep indicates that there is a problem. When this happens the nurse can reposition the wristband in front of the bar code reader or wipe the bar code reader to remove any dust that may be blocking the scan.

The other sign that there is a scanning problem is by looking at the charting software. If after scanning the bar code the patient's chart doesn't appear or the wrong chart appears, then the nurse knows there is a problem reading the patient's bar code.

When this happens the nurse retrieves the patient's chart using the keyboard and then orders a new wristband for the patient.

Let's say the nurse is administering medication to Richard Blaney, and Mr. Blaney's bar code isn't read by the bar code reader. The first step is to find Mr. Blaney's chart. With McKesson's charting software the nurse selects the HED (Horizon Expert Documentation) tab and then selects Mr. Blaney from the list of patients (Figure 10.6).

The nurse should select the patient's chart using the keyboard if the bar code reader fails to read the patient's bar code.

Mr. Blaney's chart shows his medication order. From this point, the nurse continues with the workflow as described previously in this chapter.

Solved Problems

10.1   What is a cause of medication administration errors?

Miscommunication among the practitioner, the medication order, the pharmacist, and the nurse who administers the medication can lead to medication errors.

10.2   How does electronic charting software reduce medication administration errors?

Charting software reduces the opportunity for medication errors by providing a clear channel for communication among the healthcare team and by applying built-in controls to automatically enforce the five rights of medication administration.

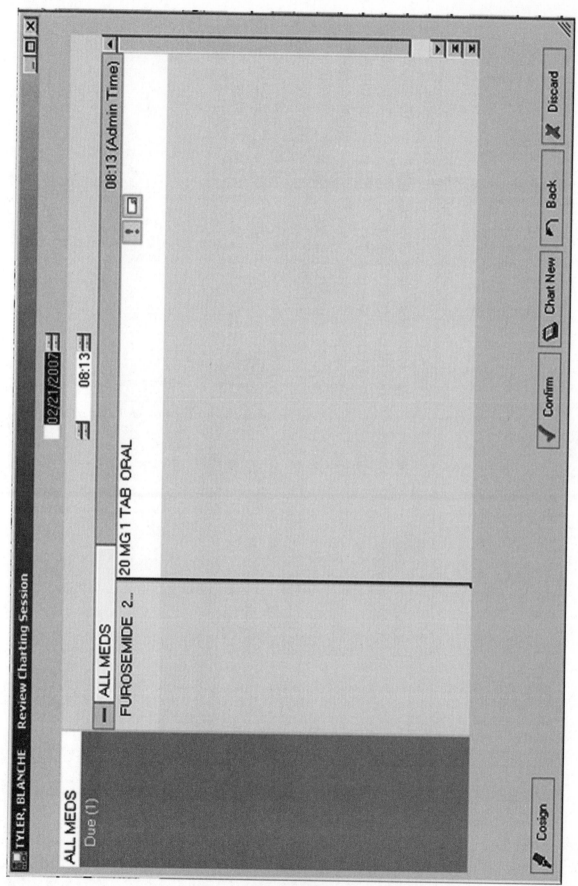

Figure 10.5

Notify	Last	First	Dept.	Rm/Bed	Diagnosis		Gen...		MRN
0	DANIELS	MELANIE	24N	2400-1	(w) ABDOMINAL PAIN UNSPEC...	Q	F	Q	000001055
1	FREMONT	LISA CAROL	24N	2401-1	(w) PATHOLOGIC FX,UNSPEC...	Q	F	Q	000001060
2	CRANE	LILA	24N	2402-1	(w) OTALGIA NOS (388.70)	Q	F	Q	000001056
3	TYLER	BLANCHE	24N	2402-2	(w) NEUROTIC DEPRESSION (...	Q	F	Q	000001065
4	DEVEREAUX	ANDRE	24N	2403-1	(w) CHEST PAIN NOS (786.50)	Q	M	Q	000001052
5	BLANEY	RICHARD	24N	2403-2	(w) FEVER (780.6)	Q	M	Q	000001051
6	LUMLEY	GEORGE	24N	2404-1	(w) CHEST PAIN NOS (786.50)	Q	M	Q	000001050
7	OACKLEY	CHARLIE	24N	2406-1	(w) GASTROINTEST HEMORR...	Q	M	Q	000001061
8	EVERGUARD	ELIZABETH	24N	2409-1	(w) TACHYCARDIA NOS (785.0)	Q	F	Q	000001121
9									

Figure 10.6

10.3   What are the five rights of medication administration?

- The right medication is administered

- To the right patient

- At the right time

- In the right dose

- Using the right route

10.4   How is the patient identified to electronic charting software?

Scanning the bar code on the patient's wristband identifies the patient.

10.5   How is the medication identified to electronic charting software?

Scanning the bar code on the medication label identifies the medication.

10.6   What should be done before scanning the patient's bar code?

The nurse must verify the identity of the patient typically by asking the patient's name and date of birth and comparing that information to the wristband. Information on the wristband may not be correct.

10.7   How is a bar code scanned?

A handheld bar code reader that is attached to the computer is placed over the patient's wristband (Figure 10.1). Pressing the button on the bar code reader causes a red light to shine on the wrist band, which reads the bar code and beeps when it is finished reading it.

10.8   What happens inside the charting software after the patient and the medication bar codes are scanned?

- The current date and time are compared to the date and time that medication is scheduled to be administered.

- The medication is compared to medications that were already administered to the patient.

- The medication, dose, and route are compared to the medication order written by the practitioner to determine if the medication that is at bedside conforms to the medication order.

- The medication is compared to other medications that the patient was recently administered to identify contraindications.

10.9   What happens if the charting software detects a violation of the five rights of medication administration?

A warning message is displayed.

10.10   What happens if the charting software does not detect a violation of the five rights of medication administration?

If no violations occur, then the charting software automatically displays that the medication was administered to the patient.

10.11   What is the first step in the medication administration workflow?

The first step is to review the medication order.

10.12   What does the nurse do if the patient refuses the medication?

The nurse selects the envelope icon in the upper-right corner to display a notepad where he can enter a comment.

10.13   What does it mean if there is no audible beep after scanning a bar code?

The scanner failed to read the bar code.

10.14   Why would a scanner fail to read a bar code on the patient's wristband?

Typically a scanner fails because the patient's wristband is damaged.

10.15   What should the nurse do if she doesn't hear a beep after scanning a bar code?

The nurse should wipe the plastic lens to remove any dust that may block the scanning and reposition the wristband or medication label in front of the bar code reader.

10.16   Why might the charting software not display the patient's chart after the patient's wristband is scanned?

This is a sign that the scanner did not properly read the bar code.

10.17   What should the nurse do if the scanner does not read the bar code even after cleaning the lens and repositioning the scanner?

The nurse must retrieve the patient's chart using the keyboard and then order a new wristband for the patient.

10.18   What happens after the nurse rescans the patient's bar code following administration of the medication?

After scanning the medication's bar code again, the charting software displays a preview of information that will be recorded in the patient's chart. This reflects any changes that the nurse made to the entry in the previous screen.

10.19   What occurs after the bar code on the medication label is scanned?

Fields are displayed to record medication administration. The number and types of fields that are available to document the medication administration vary depending on the nature of the medication and the medication order.

10.20   What should the nurse do if the number of tablets of medication on hand differs from the number of tablets displayed on the electronic chart?

The nurse can overwrite the dose and number of tablets because the pharmacy may have delivered a different dose per tablet.

10.21   Why might some charting software require that a medication's bar code be scanned twice during medication administration?

Some charting software may require that the medication bar code be scanned twice as a check and balance to assure that the medication is correct for the patient per the medication order.

10.22 Can charting software prevent all medication administration errors?

No. Charting software verifies that that the medication rights are not violated based on information in the charting software. The information in the charting software might be inaccurate. For example, the nurse might not administer the medication once it was documented that the medication was administered.

10.23 What occurs on the screen if the time to administer the medication has passed?

The charting software indicates that the medication is overdue.

10.24 Name one way charting software prevents a medication administration error?

The medication is compared to medications that were already administered to the patient. This determines if the patient already received the scheduled medication and thereby prevents the patient from receiving a second dose.

10.25 What should the nurse do if she sees a medication displayed as overdue?

She should assess the reason that the medication was not administered on time. For example, the practitioner might have issued a verbal hold order that has yet to been entered into the charting software.

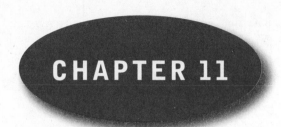

CHAPTER 11

Entering Orders

11.1 Define Order

When a patient feels something is wrong with his health, the patient visits the practitioner and reports symptoms, which are the patient's perception of what is wrong. It is up to the practitioner and the healthcare team to explore signs of disease or a disorder, which are objective findings.

This exploration usually requires medical tests. A medical test can involve analyzing bodily fluid or looking inside the patient using x-rays, magnetic resonance imaging (MRI), or, in extreme situations, a biopsy.

The practitioner writes an order directing the healthcare team to perform medical tests. Test results are additional clues to help the healthcare team diagnose the patient's problem.

Following the diagnosis the practitioner determines a course of treatment. Treatment may involve medication, therapy, or surgery. The practitioner writes an order directing the healthcare team to treat the patient.

11.1.1 Standing Order

A standing order is a medical order written in advance of the patient reporting symptoms and is executed by the healthcare team if specific signs and symptoms occur. A member of the healthcare team, who is usually a nurse, assesses the patient and determines if signs and symptoms comply with the standing order. If so, then the standing order is carried out without discussing the patient's condition and order with the practitioner.

For example, there may be a standing order for a pregnancy test for female patients who are in their childbearing years when the patient is admitted and before medication is administered. The nurse assesses the patient's age and then carries out this standing order.

Likewise, patients admitted to the healthcare facility are administered a PPD test to determine if the patient might have been exposed to TB. This test is performed based on a standing order. Also, an x-ray is ordered if the nurse determines the result of the PPD test is positive. This, too, is based on a standing order.

11.2 Entering an Electronic Order

Medical orders are entered into an electronic medical records system or a specialized system called a computerized physician order entry system (CPOE). Practitioners and other authorized members of the healthcare team can enter orders into the system. Although practitioners write the medical orders, a nurse or others on the healthcare team can enter the orders into the system.

First display the patient's chart by selecting the patient's name from the census. This is similar to other charting software.

Let's select Blanche Tyler as the patient. The charting software displays a listing of current orders for this patient (Figure 11.1). At the top of the screen is the New Order button. Select it to enter a new order for the patient.

There are hundreds of different kinds of medical orders that can be written for a patient. Charting software provides a list of these medical orders to choose from. Various techniques are used to make it easy to find the medical order.

Selecting the New Order button displays the Order Selection screen. The Order Selection screen is used to locate the type of medical order. Orders are aggregated into an order group. The order group is assigned a code. A trick to quickly finding a medical order is to know the code of the order group that contains the order.

An order group is a collection of related orders such as lab, dietary, and radiology. Depending on the charting software, groups are defined by either the software manufacturer or by the healthcare facility, which is the case with McKesson's charting software.

Each order group is assigned a code such as:

CONS = Consult

DYT = Dietary

ED = Education

LAB = Lab

NSG = Nursing

RAD = Radiology

WEIG = Weight

The group code is also referred to as an alias. The healthcare provider can enter the name of the order or the group code in the Search by box in the upper-left corner of the Order Selection screen or simply click the group in the Search Categories box. By selecting the Find button, the charting software displays a list of orders that are associated with that order group.

Let's say that Blanche Tyler's practitioner asked the nurse to enter a medical order to weigh Ms. Tyler daily. This order is in the order group identified by WEIG order group code for weight-related orders. Enter WEIG into the Search by box and click Find. The list of weight orders appears in the Order Options box (Figure 11.2).

Four medical orders are listed in the weight group. A vertical scroll bar appears if there were more medical orders than can be displayed in the Order Options box. This enables the nurse to scroll down the list.

The nurse highlights the order and clicks the Select button to copy the order to the Selected Orders box. The Selected Orders box lists the types of medical orders that nurse writes.

More than one medical order can be selected from the list by holding down the Ctrl button when highlighting the medical order.

11.2.1   Identify the Source

Identify the Order Source by entering the source in the top right corner of the Order Selection screen. The Order Source describes how the medical order is communicated. The nurse selects the Order Source from the Order Source drop-down list.

There are four types of order sources:

11.2.1.1   Written

A written medical order is a medical order that is literally written by a practitioner in the patient's paper chart. This occurs during the period when the healthcare facility is transitioning from paper to electronic charts. The written medical order must be transcribed into the electronic order.

OE - Current Orders - TYLER, BLANCHE - 2402-2

Patient View Setup Order Guidelines Mgr Help

Privacy   Allergy

Action Items   Primary CD: (None)   Current Phase: (None)

New Order... Sched... Actions... Variances... Phase Mgr...
Review... Results... Change... Discontinue/Correct... Hold...

Group	Description	Num	Status	Pending Actions	Order DT/TM	Start Date	End Date
DTY	LOW TRIGLYCERIDE MEALS DTY TIMED	0013	Ordered		04/26/06 1304	04/26/06 1304	
DTYS	HIGH FIBER MEALS DTY TIMED	0012	Ordered		04/26/06 1259	04/26/06 1259	
LAB	CULTURE, BLOOD ONCE ROUTINE	0010 (0008	Active		04/25/06 1841	04/25/06 1903	04/25/06 1903
	CULTURE, BLOOD STAT x1 Occurrence STAT	0009 (0008	Active		04/25/06 1841	04/25/06 1840	04/25/06 1840
NSG	IF TEMP > 101 PRN PRN	0011	Partial		04/25/06 1842	04/24/06 1839	
PAN	BLOOD CULTURES X2 ONCE ROUTINE	0008 (P)	Active		04/25/06 1841	04/25/06 1839	04/25/06 1839

Figure 11.1

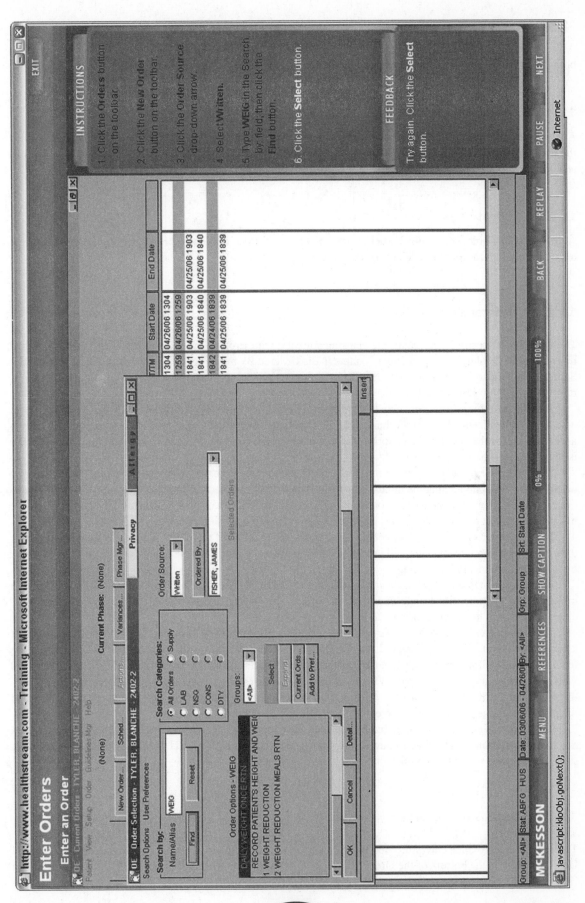

Figure 11.2

11.2.1.2 Verbal

A verbal medical order is a medical order told to the nurse by the practitioner. This commonly occurs when both the practitioner and the nurse are at the patient's bedside during daily rounds.

11.2.1.3 Telephone

A telephone medical order is similar to a verbal medical order except that the practitioner calls the nurse to relay the medical order. This happens frequently when the nurse calls the practitioner to report results of a medical test and the practitioner orders a follow-up test or treatment.

11.2.1.4 Direct

A direct medical order is a medical order entered by the practitioner or the authorized member of the healthcare team directly into the electronic charting software.

11.2.2 Ordered By

The nurse must specify in the electronic charting software who wrote the medical order. This is accomplished by entering the healthcare team member's name in the Ordered By box. The Ordered By box is below the Order Source box in the top right corner of the Order Selection screen. Some charting software, including McKesson's, refer to the person who writes the order as the provider.

A drop-down list of providers may be displayed. The drop-down list typically lists the patient's practitioners who have written medical orders for the patient. Furthermore, the patient's primary practitioner might be chosen as the default for the new order and appear automatically in the Ordered By box. In this example, James Fisher is Ms. Tyler's primary practitioner.

Listing the default practitioner automatically into the Ordered By box is a timesaving feature but is also risky because an assumption is that the default practitioner is writing the medical order. However, a different practitioner might have written the medical order. It is because of this risk that some healthcare facilities may choose not to set a default practitioner or a list of practitioners who most frequently write orders for the patient.

If the provider's name doesn't appear in the drop-down list box or if there isn't a list or default provider, then the nurse must search from among all practitioners who are associated with the healthcare facility. This is done by clicking the Ordered By button.

Selecting the Ordered By button causes the Staff Select screen to appear (Figure 11.3). This is where the nurse locates the practitioner who is writing the order. This is like finding a needle in a haystack; however, charting software has a few shortcuts to make the search easier.

The search can be limited to a particular group of staff by selecting from the Group drop-down list that appears on the left side of the screen. Likewise, the nurse can limit the search to a specific facility by picking from the Facility drop-down list located below the Group drop-down list.

The nurse enters the full or partial name of the provider in the box at the top of the screen and then clicks the Find button. The charting software displays every staff member that matches the search criteria. The nurse highlights the name and selects OK to enter the provider in the order.

If the nurse is unsure of spelling, but he can spell the name phonetically, he selects the Soundex box, enters the phonetic spelling of the practitioner in the search criteria, and then selects the Find button. The charting software searches the staff for names that match the search criteria.

11.2.3 Details of the Order

The healthcare provider enters the details of the order once the medical order is selected. She selects the Details button on the bottom of the Order Selection screen. The Details button opens the Order Detail screen (Figure 11.4).

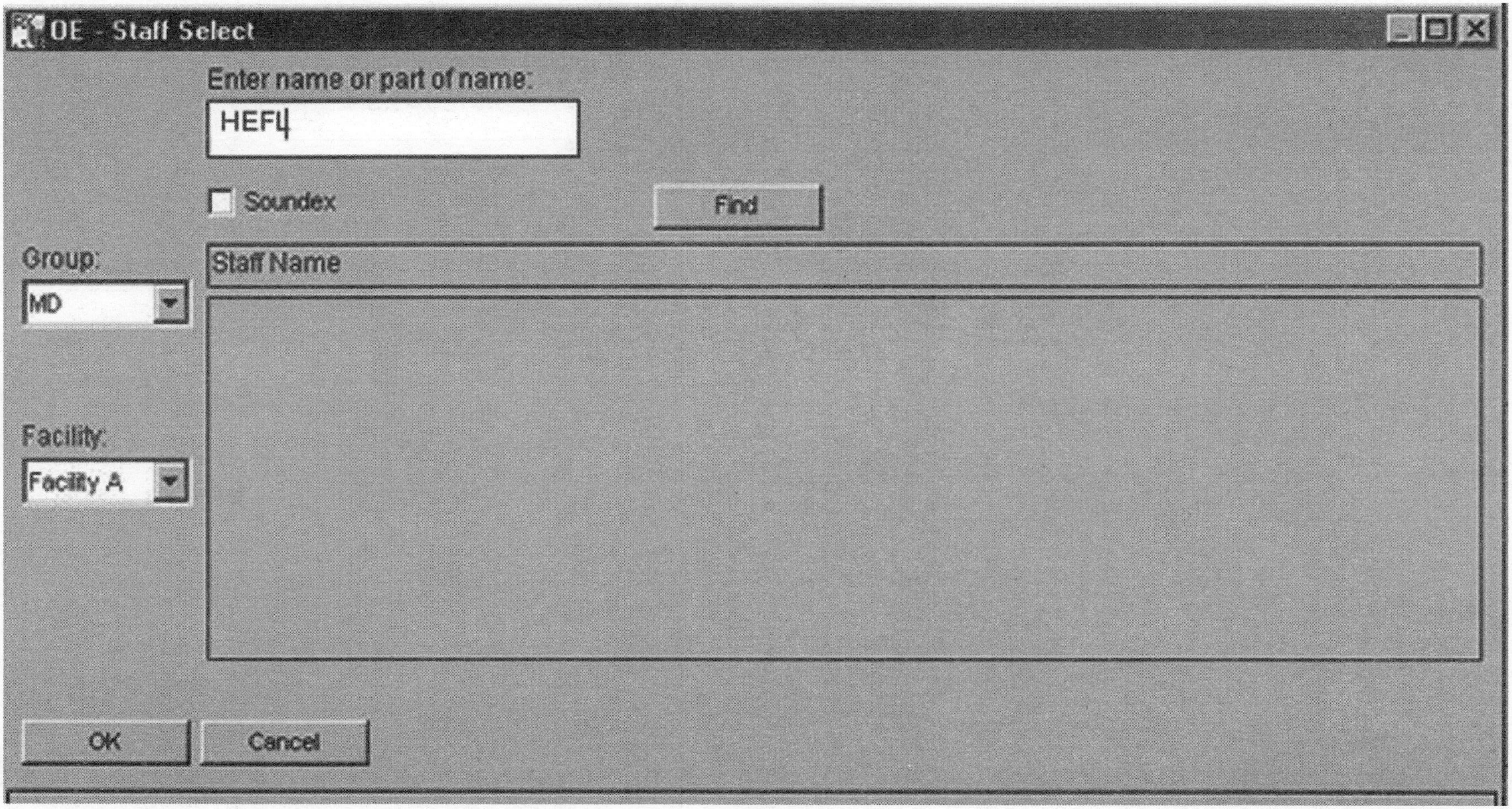

Figure 11.3

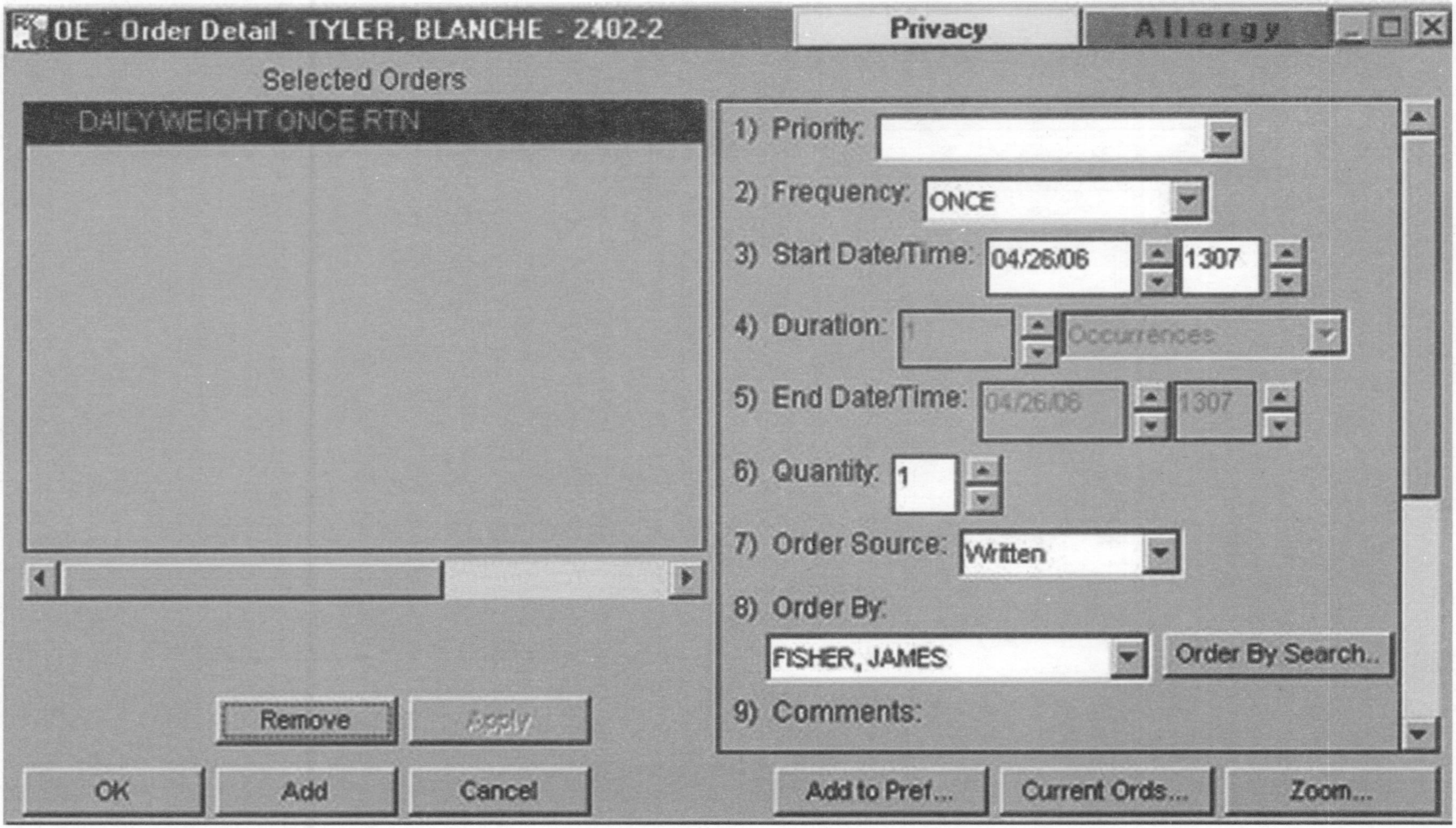

OE - Order Detail - TYLER, BLANCHE - 2402-2

Privacy   Allergy

Selected Orders

DAILY WEIGHT ONCE RTN

1) Priority:

2) Frequency: ONCE

3) Start Date/Time: 04/26/06   1307

4) Duration: Occurrences

5) End Date/Time: 04/26/06   1307

6) Quantity: 1

7) Order Source: Written

8) Order By:
   FISHER, JAMES

9) Comments:

Order By Search...

Remove   Apply

OK   Add   Cancel   Add to Pref...   Current Ords...   Zoom...

164

Figure 11.4

The Order Detail screen displays a list of selected medical orders on the right side of the screen. In this example, there is one medical order, which is daily weight for Ms. Tyler. Additional orders would appear if multiple medical orders were selected.

Highlighting the medical order causes the charting software to display details that are associated with the order. Details will differ depending on the nature of the medical order.

Some details such as start date and time and frequency are already filled in. These are default settings. The nurse must verify that these settings are correct and change them if necessary.

Other details are blank, requiring the nurse to enter information. This can be accomplished by selecting a choice from a drop-down menu or using up and down arrows to change the value displayed on the screen, as is the case with Quantity.

Still other details are grayed, prohibiting the nurse from changing the value. Charting software grays a value for one of three reasons:

- The value cannot be changed until the nurse enter a previous value. Once the previous value is entered, charting software ungrays the value, enabling the nurse to change it.

- The value is set by default. For example, if frequency is set to Once, the duration must be 1.

- The detail does not pertain to the order.

The nurse can select the Remove button on the Order Detail screen to remove the medical order. The Add button is used to insert a new medical order. Selecting OK saves the order to the patient's chart.

11.3   Compound Medical Order

A compound order is a medical order that consists of two or more other medical orders and is identified by a unique name. A complete blood count (CBC) is an example. CBC is a group of blood tests that are commonly ordered together to provide the healthcare team with a glimpse into the patient's health.

The healthcare facility or the charting software manufacturer defines groups of tests based on the policy of the healthcare facility and defines the group code, or alias, to the compound order. Enter the group code, or alias, as the search criteria to display the compound order.

Once the compound medical order is selected, the charting software compares medical orders that make up the compound medical order with medical orders already written for the patient in an effort to prevent duplicate orders from being entered.

For example, a practitioner may have previously written a medical order for a white blood count (WBC) to determine if the patient has an infection. Subsequently, an order might be written for a CBC, which is a compound order that includes a WBC.

Rather than automatically processing the CBC order, the charting software searches previous orders to determine if the WBC had been ordered. If so, depending on the type of charting software being used, the charting software either removes the WBC from the CBC order or enters a comment on the CBC order that the WBC was already ordered.

11.4   Computerized Physician Order Entry

Many healthcare facilities use a computerized physician order entry system (CPOE) that enables physicians and other prescribers to enter medical orders electronically. CPOE orders replace orders written by prescribers on paper, although the process of taking off orders is still necessary.

When a paper order is written, the prescriber "flags" the order by inserting the last two hole punches in the paper order into the first two rings in the paper chart causing the top part of the paper order to extend beyond the top of the chart. The physician may also turn a wheel on the spin of the chart exposing the color yellow or red. Yellow indicates that an order was taken off and is ready to be cosigned, and red implies that the order has not been taken off and the order requires immediate attention. The prescriber then places the chart back on the rack.

The nurse realizes there is a pending order by scanning the color wheel on the spine of the chart. The nurse processes a pending order using the procedure called "taking off orders." This procedure requires the nurse to read and execute the order. The process of executing the order depends on the nature of the order. Medication orders are typically faxed to the pharmacy and entered into the medication record administration (MAR) book. Lab and imagining orders are either faxed to the appropriate department or the department is called. Orders that can be carried out by the nurse are executed immediately.

Once orders are taken off, the color wheel is turned to yellow indicating that another nurse needs to verify the order and check that the order was taken off properly. This is referred as cosigning the order. The goal is to ensure that no errors occur and that the order was correctly transcribed to the MAR. The color wheel is turned to green once the order is cosigned.

11.4.1 Processing CPOE Orders

CPOE orders are electronically entered by the prescriber, eliminating the need for the prescriber to write a paper order. There are two exceptions: when the CPOE system does not have elements of the order or if the healthcare facility's policies prohibit CPOE orders. The CPOE system contains all items that a prescriber can order when the CPOE system is implemented. However, there may be a lag between when a healthcare facility acquires new items and when those new items are available in the CPOE system. During this lag period, prescribers use paper orders to request those items.

The healthcare facility can institute policies that require some procedures to be excluded from the CPOE system in order to preserve privacy for the patient such as in the case of an HIV test. Although access to the CPOE system and other elements of the electronic medical records is controlled by ID and password, there is always the possibility that the data can be hacked, enabling unauthorized access to patient data. The healthcare facility balances the benefits of having electronic patient information against the risk of unauthorized access of the data. In situations where the risk is high, the healthcare facility records the data on paper.

For example, an HIV test is ordered on paper, and the results are placed in a sealed envelope. The nurse or the prescriber must pick up the envelope personally at the lab, thereby reducing the chance that the information will fall into unauthorized hands.

After the prescriber enters a CPOE order, a yellow square appears on the unit's census in the work queue (WQ) column (Figure 11.5) indicating that there is a pending order. An uncolored square in the WQ column indicates there are no pending orders.

Double clicking the yellow square displays a list of orders for that patient in the Order Manager Work queue screen (Figure 11.6). The Order Manager Work queue screen is divided into three sections. The top contains a list of patients. The patient that is selected is highlighted on the list. The healthcare provider can also select other patients on the list to view their pending orders. This saves time from going back to the census to process other orders.

The center section of the Order Manager Work queue screen contains two tabs. These are the CPOE OM Orders and CPOE Rx Orders. The CPOE OM Orders tab contains non-medication orders. The CPOE Rx Orders tab contains only medication orders. Nurses are able to take off CPOE OM Orders. The pharmacy takes off CPOE Rx Orders.

The CPOE OM Orders tab lists CPOE orders that the prescriber entered. Highlighting the order causes details of the order to be displayed in the lower portion of the Order Manager Work queue screen. The healthcare facility's policy requires that orders be processed within a specific time period, which is tracked by the CPOE software. If that time period has expired, the CPOE software displays the overdue message.

Some orders are displayed with a plus sign. This indicates that the prescriber entered a group of orders. Group orders are common when the patient is to undergo a routine procedure. In this example, the patient is being admitted and requires routine admission orders. Other information in the center portion of the screen provides a brief description of the order.

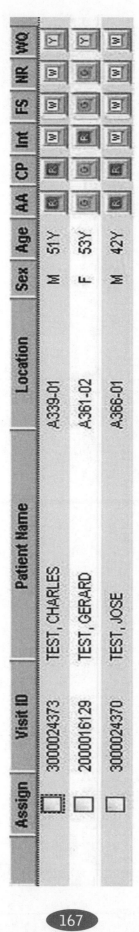

Figure 11.5

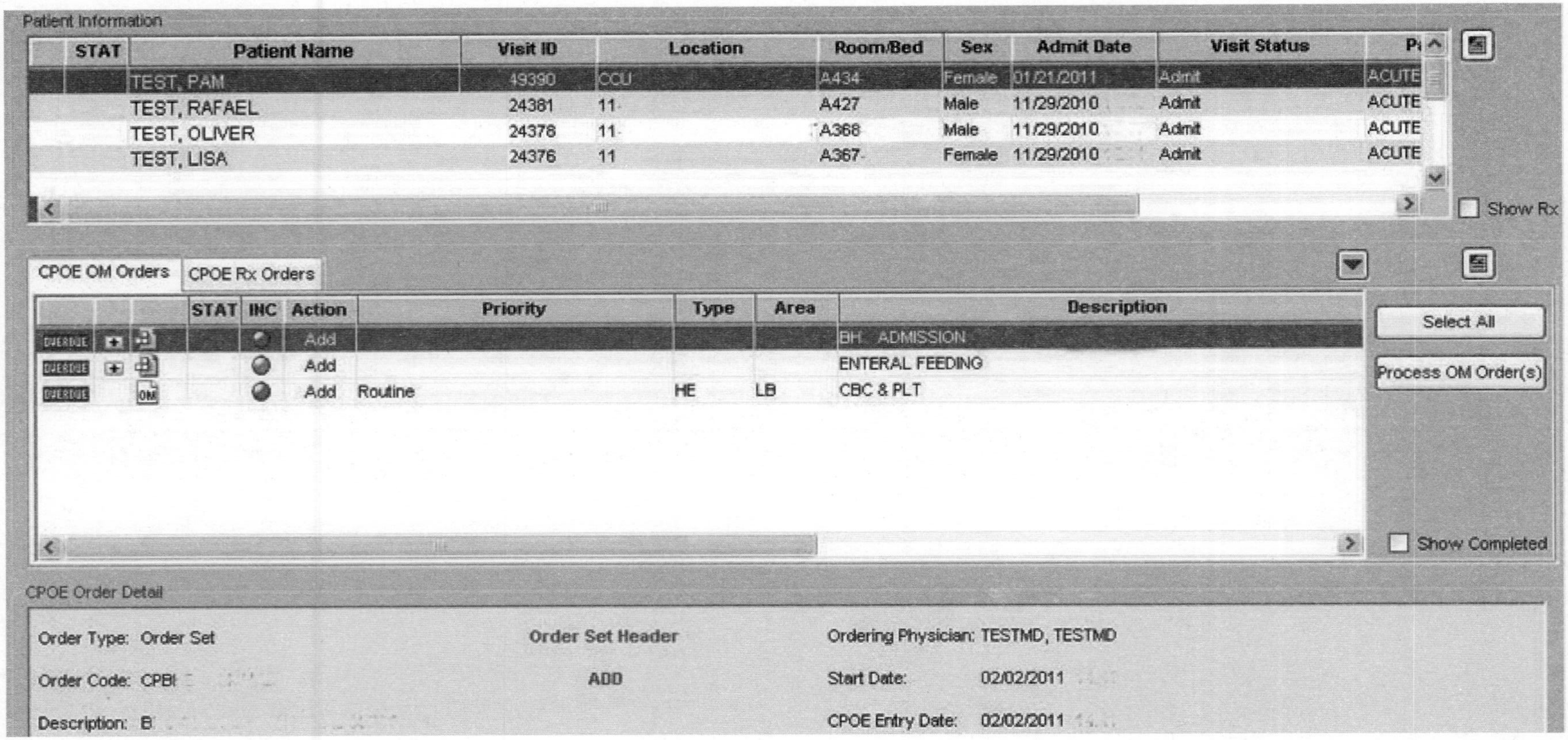
Patient Information
STAT
Patient Name
Visit ID
Location
Room/Bed
Sex
Admit Date
Visit Status
TEST, PAM 49390 CCU A434 Female 01/21/2011 Admit ACUTE
TEST, RAFAEL 24381 11 A427 Male 11/29/2010 Admit ACUTE
TEST, OLIVER 24378 11 A368 Male 11/29/2010 Admit ACUTE
TEST, LISA 24376 11 A367 Female 11/29/2010 Admit ACUTE
Show Rx
CPOE OM Orders
CPOE Rx Orders
STAT
INC
Action
Priority
Type
Area
Description
Add BH ADMISSION
Add ENTERAL FEEDING
Add Routine HE LB CBC & PLT
Select All
Process OM Order(s)
Show Completed
CPOE Order Detail
Order Type: Order Set
Order Set Header
Ordering Physician: TESTMD, TESTMD
Order Code: CPBI
ADD
Start Date: 02/02/2011
Description: B
CPOE Entry Date: 02/02/2011

Figure 11.6

The nurse must take off orders in the CPOE OM Orders tab by highlighting the order and selecting the Process OM Order(s) button. Alternatively the nurse can select the Select All button to process all the pending orders on this tab for the patient. Once orders are processed, the yellow box in the WQ column turns white. However, the box may remain yellow after the nurse has processed the patient's CPOE OM Orders if the pharmacy has yet to take off the medication orders.

11.4.2   Taking Off CPOE Orders

When the Process OM Order(s) button is selected, the Order Entry screen is automatically displayed (Figure 11.7). If the order is a single order, then basic information about the order is displayed. If the order is a group order, then a list of orders that comprise the group is displayed in a box with the first order in the group highlighted and displayed on the screen.

Some orders are complete when written by the prescriber. In those situations, the nurse reviews the order and selects OK to process the order. The nurse has the option to correct any errors on the order before the order is processed.

CPOE orders are not necessarily complete when written, which is very similar to paper orders, because the prescriber lacks all the information to process the order. For example, the prescriber may order medication be administered three times a day on the next schedule. The healthcare facility's policy specifies the actual times when three-times-a-day medication is administered. The pharmacist who takes off the medication order schedules the medication in the MAR according to the healthcare facility's policy.

Likewise, the prescriber may order a GI consult for the patient but does not know when the consulting physician is available. The nurse may be expected to call the consulting physician and schedule the consult then enter the date as the Start Date for the order.

If the order is part of a group order, the processed order is removed from the list of pending orders and the next order on the list is displayed. The healthcare provider can select the Skip button or simply highlight a different order on the list if he chooses not to process the order now. Skipping an order is commonly done when some of the information necessary to process the order is lacking. The healthcare provider can process other orders in the group of orders and then return later to process the remaining pending order. The WQ box remains yellow as long as at least one order is pending so that the nurse will not forget that there is a pending order.

11.4.3   Confirmation Orders

It might seem that electronic medical records would replace paper medical records. This is not the case. Many healthcare facilities continue with some form of a paper medical record that is used as a backup in case computers are not available. This is also true with CPOE orders.

After the nurse or pharmacist takes off a CPOE order, the CPOE system processes the order electronically and prints a confirmation of the order. Depending on the healthcare facility's policy, the department who is carrying out the order receives both an electronic and print notification of the order and the unit where the patient resides receives a printed confirmation of all processed orders.

Figure 11.8 illustrates the printed confirmation of medication orders. Confirmations are usually printed in the unit's medication room to ensure privacy and to prevent the confirmation from being inadvertently removed from a printer used to print other documents on the unit.

Printed confirmation of orders is placed in the Physician Order section of the patient's paper chart. Confirmation of medication orders are also used to update the MAR in healthcare facilities that do not use an electronic MAR. In this situation, the nurse manually enters the medication into the MAR and another nurse cosigns the entry ensuring that the transcription is correct.

For new patients, the printed MAR contains medication orders that the prescriber ordered as part of admission orders and therefore the nurse does not need to transcribe the medication order to the MAR. However, the nurse still must cosign the order to ensure that the MAR contains medication orders that the prescriber ordered.

For existing patients, the printed MAR is reprinted once a week, at which time the nurse must compare the updated existing MAR to the newly printed MAR to ensure accuracy.

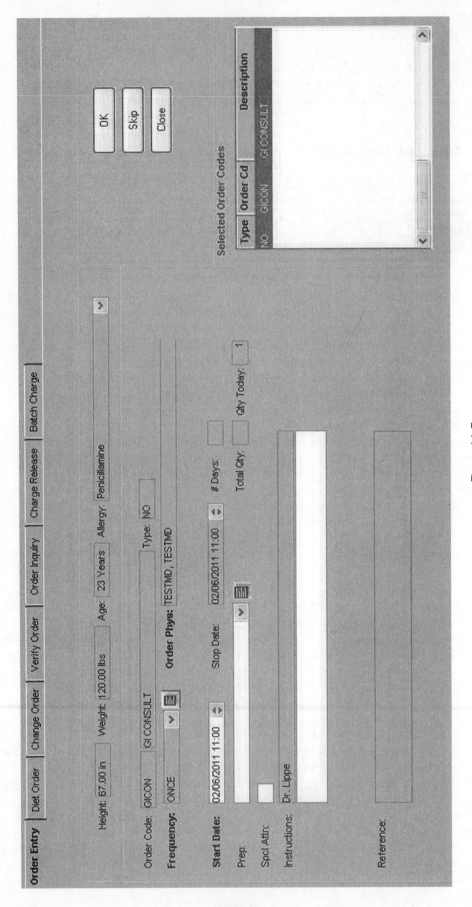

Figure 11.7

PAT NAME: TEST, PAM
N/S: CCU Room/Bed: A43.
SEX: Female DOB: 08/16/2007 Age: 3Y
Allergies: Acetadote
Working Diagnosis:
ATTEND PHY: TESTMD, TESTMD

Action	CPOE#	Ord#/RX#	Order Desc	Dose	Route	Freq/Rate	Priority	Duration	Start	Stop
Add	2813		THIAMINE HCL TABLET	100 MG	PO	ONCE A DAY			Next Sch. Time	

Description	Dose	UOM	Frequency
Meds THIAMINE HCL TABLET	100	MG	

Action	CPOE#	Ord#/RX#	Order Desc	Dose	Route	Freq/Rate	Priority	Duration	Start	Stop
Add	2814		FOLIC ACID TABLET	1 MG	PO	ONCE A DAY			Next Sch. Time	

Description	Dose	UOM	Frequency
Meds FOLIC ACID TABLET	1	MG	

Action	CPOE#	Ord#/RX#	Order Desc	Dose	Route	Freq/Rate	Priority	Duration	Start	Stop
Add	2815		MULTIVITAMIN CAPSULE	1 CAPSULE	PO	ONCE A DAY			Next Sch. Time	

Description	Dose	UOM	Frequency
Meds MULTIVITAMIN CAPSULE	1	CAPSULE	

Action	CPOE#	Ord#/RX#	Order Desc	Dose	Route	Freq/Rate	Priority	Duration	Start	Stop
Add	2816		NICOTINE 14MG PATCH PATCH EVERY 24	1 PATCH	TD	ONCE A DAY			Next Sch. Time	

Figure 11.8

11.5   Dietary Orders

Clinicians write dietary orders based on the patient's nutritional requirements. Before a dietary order is written, a dietician assesses the patient and documents the assessment in the Diet tab of the patient's Daily Focus Assessment (Figure 11.9). The dietary assessment determines the patient's feeding ability and if the patient has difficulty chewing or swallowing. In addition, the dietician identifies if the patient is on a tube feeding and, if so, the nature of the tube feeding, i.e., NG tube or G tube.

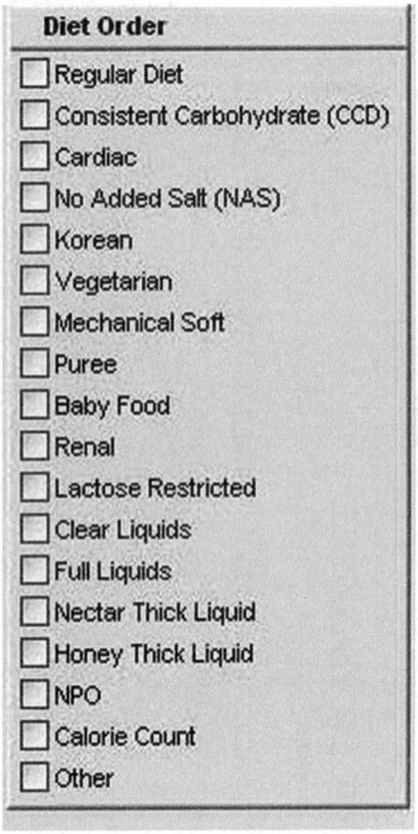

Diet Order

- [ ] Regular Diet
- [ ] Consistent Carbohydrate (CCD)
- [ ] Cardiac
- [ ] No Added Salt (NAS)
- [ ] Korean
- [ ] Vegetarian
- [ ] Mechanical Soft
- [ ] Puree
- [ ] Baby Food
- [ ] Renal
- [ ] Lactose Restricted
- [ ] Clear Liquids
- [ ] Full Liquids
- [ ] Nectar Thick Liquid
- [ ] Honey Thick Liquid
- [ ] NPO
- [ ] Calorie Count
- [ ] Other

Figure 11.9

The dietician determines the number of calories and protein per day that the patient should receive and the diet order. The diet order specifies if the patient is on a regular diet, no-added-salt diet for hypertension, consistent carbohydrate diet for diabetes, or other special diets.

Although the dietician documents the diet order in the Diet tab of the Daily Focus Assessment, the diet order must be submitted by the practitioner. Depending on the policy of the healthcare facility, the diet order can only be written by a prescriber. The dietician can assess the patient's dietary needs and recommend to the prescriber a diet for the patient; however the dietician cannot write the diet order.

The diet order is written by the prescriber using the CPOE or on paper. The order is then processed by the nurse. The diet order screen appears when the CPOE order is processed. If the order is on paper, the nurse must manually display the diet order screen by selecting an icon on the toolbar to open the order system.

The diet order screen (Figure 11.10) lists available diets. There is an item on the list called Special Diets that when selected enables the nurse to enter dietary options that are not listed. The nurse elects the diet from the list. The diet order then appears in the lower portion of the screen. The start date and time default to the date and time that the order was entered. The stop date and time default to zero implying that the diet continues throughout the patient's stay on the unit. The nurse can change the date and time, and the dietary department will deliver the diet according to those changes.

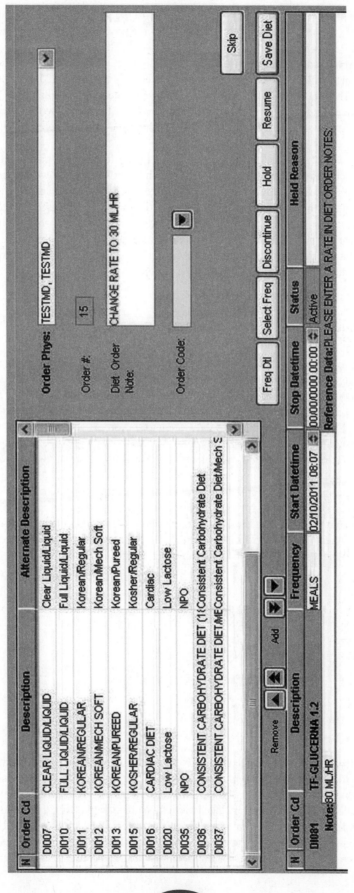

Figure 11.10

The nurse needs to enter the frequency of the diet. By default, the order is carried out for every meal. The nurse can specify alternative times such as between meals or breakfast only depending on the prescriber's directions.

Probably the most frequently used feature of the diet order screen is the diet order note. The diet order note is a free-form comment that allows the dietary department to modify the standard dietary order that was selected from the list of diets. The diet order note is also where the nurse enters the patient's likes and dislikes of foods.

For example, the patient may prefer non-pork products so the nurse would write a diet-order note saying, "no pork." Likewise, the patient may like pasta without red sauce. Therefore, the nurse would write, "no red sauce."

Depending on the healthcare facility's policy, the nurse is able to enter the patient's likes and dislikes into an existing dietary order without consulting the prescriber and the dietician. However, the nurse is not permitted to materially change the diet order. For example, the nurse cannot change a cardiac diet to a regular diet.

There are times when the healthcare facility expects the nurse to act based on the best interest of the patient. For example, a new patient arrives on the unit and is diagnosed with hypertension. The prescriber orders a regular diet for the patient an hour or so before meals are served. If the nurse is unable to contact the prescriber for clarification, depending on the healthcare faciliy's policy the nurse is expected to change the dietary order to "no added salt" in order to protect the patient.

11.6 Orders Inquiry and Changing Orders

The healthcare provider can inquire about any order entered into the system by selecting the patient from the census list and opening the electronic orders system. He selects the Order Inquiry tab. Orders are listed in a table. Each row is an order, and columns represent characteristics of the order. The list can be rearranged by selecting the column name. This causes the orders to be sorted according to the value in the column name. For example, selecting the Start Date column causes the system to sort orders according to Start Date. Select it once for descending and a second time for ascending order.

It is also useful to sort by description to compare the results of the same test over a period of time. The system then lists the same tests in the same area of the list of orders.

Icons are used to indicate that the nurse should review the results of the order. An "i" icon indicates results are normal but have yet to be reviewed. An exclamation icon indicates an abnormal value. A red "C" icon indicates a critical value (Figure 11.11). The lab usually calls the unit if there is a critical value. Boxes appear in the first column of orders when results have not been reviewed. The nurse is expected to select each box indicating that he or she reviewed the results. Double clicking an order enables the nurse to view details of the order.

ⓘ	5 HCGS	UA	HCG PREGNANCY TEST SERUM
▲	4 CBCD	HE	CBC & DIFF & PLT
▲	3 CMP	CH	P14 /INCLUDES HFP
Ⓒ	2 ALCS	CH	ALCOHOL SERUM

Figure 11.11

An order can be changed by selecting the Change Order tab. The Change Order tab contains a list of orders. The nurse highlights the order she wants changed and then selects the Update Status. By default, No Update is the selected status. The other options are Discontinue, Cancel, or Reinstate the order (Figure 11.12).

Discontinue is selected when the order has been carried out and the prescriber wants to stop the order before the Stop Date of the order. The Stop Date is a component of the order. The Cancel order is selected when the order has not been carried out as of yet. The Reinstate status is used to reverse a discontinued or cancelled order without having to re-enter the order into the system. Once the Update Status is entered, the nurse selects the Execute button to process the change.

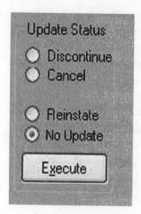

Figure 11.12

The Change Order tab doesn't allow the nurse to actually modify the original order. In essence, he terminates the original order and starts over with a new order rather than altering details of the original order. This is a safety measure to prevent errors from occurring when changing an order. In addition, this separates orders. That is, the existing order is no longer valid. The modification is actually a new order.

11.7 Response to Orders

Once the order is processed, the nurse must ensure that the order is carried out. Some orders, such as inserting an NG tube, are carried out by the nurse. Other orders are carried out by other members of the patient's healthcare team, such as the lab technician. Regardless of who carries out the order, the outcome of the order must be documented in the patient's electronic chart.

For example, medication orders are processed by the pharmacy and carried out by the nurse when medication is administered to the patient. Medication administration is noted in the electronic medical administration record (EMAR). However, PRN medications are also noted in the Daily Focus Assessment. Administering a PRN medication is an exception to the patient's scheduled treatment plan and needs to be called to the clinician's attention by entering the PRN in the electronic chart in addition to the EMAR. Prior to rounds, the clinician reviews the electronic chart for recent patient activities. The clinician does not review the EMAR.

Non-medication orders need to be documented in the electronic chart when the order is carried out. The electronic chart usually has an area where each order is documented, which can be seen in detail in Chapter 10. Most of the time outcomes of orders are recorded in the Daily Focus Assessment.

If there isn't a place in the Daily Focus Assessment to chart the outcomes of orders, then the nurse charts the outcome in a progress note. Some nurses prefer using the progress note rather than selecting items from the Daily Focus Assessment because they feel the narrative provides a more complete description than selecting a few items from a list. However, a progress notes does not lend itself to computerized statistical analysis. Computer software can count the number of times a particular Daily Focus Assessment item was selected, but it is unable to parse the narrative in a progress note.

Abnormal and critical lab outcomes need to be documented in the patient's electronic chart using the ABN/Critical Values tab in the Daily Focus Assessment. As indicated previously in this chapter, an abnormal lab value appears as a yellow square in the NR column on the census and a critical lab value appears as a red square on the census. Selecting the square displays the lab results.

An abnormal value is a value outside the normal range as determined by the healthcare facility's lab. A critical value is also outside of the normal range, but this is so far outside the range that the patient's health may be in imminent danger. The lab calls the unit informing the nurse of the critical value. The nurse is expected to contact the clinician immediately to address the problem.

The abnormal and critical value must also be entered in the ABN/Critical Values tab in the Daily Focus Assessment (Figure 11.13). The nurse primarily documents when he was notified, who he in turn notified, and what the intervention was. Fields on the ABN/Critical Values tabs are self-explained, however the nurse should clarify the entry into the Abnormal/Critical Result text box. He enters the results in the text box and then enters a Group Note for the text box that explains the nature of the test and additional information that would help further explain the situation.

The clinician does not use documentation in the ABN/Critical Values tab to assess the patient and determine the proper intervention. The clinician reviews the actual lab results and other assessments in the patient's electronic chart to determine the proper course of action. The ABN/Critical Values tab is used by the nurse to record the notification of the abnormal or critical lab and the activities she performed to react to the notification.

11.8   Telephone Orders

Telephone orders are medical orders that the prescriber dictates to the nurse over the telephone when the prescriber is unavailable to enter the order in the CPOE system or write the order on a paper order.

CPOE systems have reduced but not eliminated the need for telephone orders because, depending on the healthcare facility's policies, prescribers are able to access the CPOE system from within the healthcare facility and remotely. Therefore, there are fewer times when the prescriber is unable to write the medical order electronically.

In reality, telephone orders remain part of daily activities on the unit for a number of reasons—primarily convenience. A typical scenario is the patient's condition has changed and the nurse notifies the prescriber by telephone. If the condition is routine and does not require the prescriber to assess the patient, then the prescriber will dictate a telephone order to the nurse. The whole interaction may last only 30 seconds. The nurse then focuses on carrying out the order.

Alternatively, the prescriber can tell the nurse that the prescriber will enter the CPOE order. This can take longer than 30 seconds, especially if the prescriber is not in front of a computer. Further delays occur if the prescriber is seeing other patients before time is available to enter the order. And, there is always the chance that the prescriber will forget to enter the order.

For example, a patient may come to the nurse's station after dinner complaining about indigestion. The patient does not have Maalox as a PRN order so the nurse calls the prescriber for a medication order for Maalox. The prescriber realizes that indigestion is likely caused by the dinner and orders Maalox 30 ml PO one time now. The fastest way to relieve the patient's indigestion is if the order is taken as a telephone order.

Telephone orders can be entered in the CPOE system, if the healthcare facility's policy grants nurses the rights to the CPOE system. Some healthcare facilities have an electronic order processing system aside from the CPOE system, which is used for processing orders rather than writing orders. The last option is for the nurse to write a paper order and fax the order to the pharmacy. The pharmacy will then send the medication to the unit or someone from the unit will pick up the medication at the pharmacy. Alternatively, some medications, such as Maalox, may be on the unit already and can be given to the patient without delay.

Solved Problems

11.1   What is a medical order?

A medical order is an instruction to the healthcare team written by a practitioner to perform a medical test or treatment on a patient.

11.2   What is a standing order?

A standing order is a medical order written in advance of the patient reporting symptoms and is executed by the healthcare team if specific signs and symptoms occur. A member of the healthcare

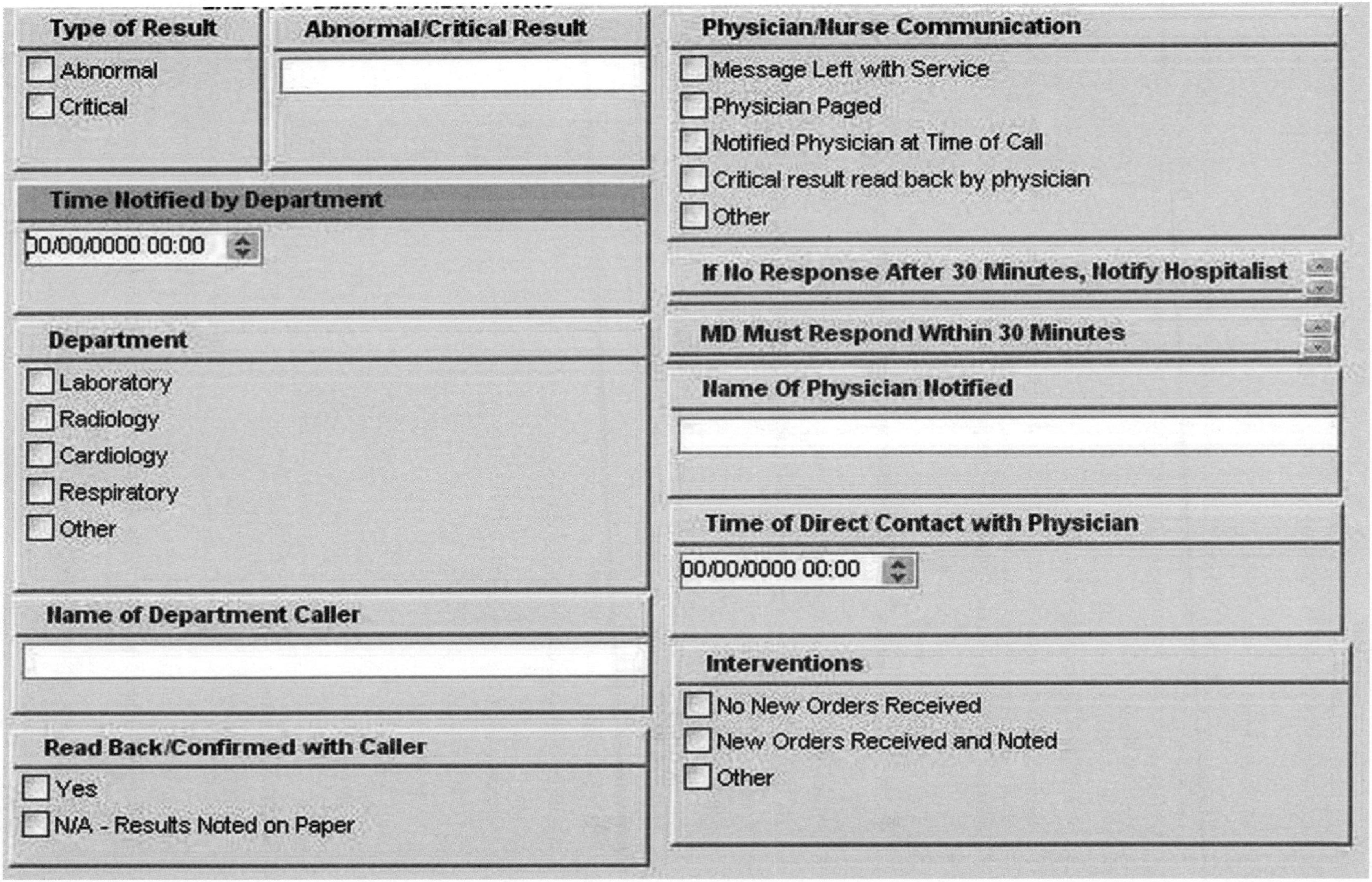

Type of Result

- ☐ Abnormal
- ☐ Critical

Abnormal/Critical Result

Time Notified by Department

00/00/0000 00:00 ◆

Department

- ☐ Laboratory
- ☐ Radiology
- ☐ Cardiology
- ☐ Respiratory
- ☐ Other

Name of Department Caller

Read Back/Confirmed with Caller

- ☐ Yes
- ☐ N/A - Results Noted on Paper

Physician/Nurse Communication

- ☐ Message Left with Service
- ☐ Physician Paged
- ☐ Notified Physician at Time of Call
- ☐ Critical result read back by physician
- ☐ Other

If No Response After 30 Minutes, Notify Hospitalist

MD Must Respond Within 30 Minutes

Name Of Physician Notified

Time of Direct Contact with Physician

00/00/0000 00:00 ◆

Interventions

- ☐ No New Orders Received
- ☐ New Orders Received and Noted
- ☐ Other

Figure 11.13

team, who is usually a nurse, assesses the patient and determines if signs and symptoms comply with the standing order. If so, then the standing order is carried out without discussing the patient's condition and order with the practitioner.

11.3 Give an example of a standing order.

Patients admitted to the healthcare facility are administered a PPD test to determine if the patient has been exposed to TB. This test is performed based on a standing order. Also, an x-ray is ordered if the nurse determines the results of the PPD test is positive. This, too, is based on a standing order

11.4 Why are medical orders written?

Medical orders are written for evaluative tests to provide objective signs of disease or disorder to the practitioner in order for the practitioner to make a medical diagnosis. Once a diagnosis is made, additional medical orders are written to treat the patient.

11.5 What is a CPOE system?

This is a computerized physician order entry system used by physicians to write medical orders.

11.6 What is the first step to entering a medical order?

The first step is to display the patient's chart by selecting the patient's name from the census.

11.7 What is an order group?

An order group is a logical aggregation of similar medical orders into a group. An order group is a collection of related orders such as lab, dietary, and radiology.

11.8 How is an order group identified?

Each order group is identified by a group code.

11.9 Give an example of a group code.

CONS = Consult

DYT = Dietary

ED = Education

LAB = Lab

NSG = Nursing

RAD = Radiology

WEIG = Weight

11.10 Who decides which medical orders are assigned to an order group?

Either the healthcare facility or the the charting software manufacturer decides.

11.11 What is the first step in the medication administration workflow?

The first step is to review the medication order.

11.12   How can the nurse select more than one medical order?

More than one medical order can be selected from the list by holding down the Ctrl button when highlighting the medical order.

11.13   What is a written medical order?

This is a medical order that is literally written by a practitioner in the patient's paper chart. This occurs during the period when the healthcare facility is transitioning from paper to electronic charts. The written medical order must be transcribed into the electronic order.

11.14   What is a verbal medical order?

A verbal medical order is a medical order told to the nurse by the practitioner. This commonly occurs when both the practitioner and the nurse are at the patient's bedside during daily rounds.

11.15   What is a telephone order?

A telephone medical order is similar to a verbal medical order except that the practitioner relays the medical order to the nurse by phone. This happens frequently when the nurse calls the practitioner to report results of a medical test, and the practitioner orders a follow-up test or treatment.

11.16   What is a direct medical order?

A direct medical order is medical order entered by the practitioner or an authorized member of the healthcare team directly into the electronic charting software.

11.17   What is the purpose of the Ordered By box?

The Ordered By box is used to identify who wrote the medical order.

11.18   Who might be listed as the default name in the Ordered By box?

The patient's primary practitioner is sometimes listed as the default name.

11.19   Who are listed in the drop-down list of practitioners in the Ordered By box?

These are practitioners who have written medical orders for the patient.

11.20   What should the nurse do if the practitioner does not appear on the Ordered By box drop-down list?

The nurse can search for the practitioner from a list of all practitioners associated with the healthcare facility.

11.21   What should the nurse do if he cannot locate the practitioner on the list of all practitioners associated with the healthcare facility?

He should contact the healthcare facility's support staff who are responsible for the electronic charting software. Typically, those members of the healthcare team who are authorized to write medical orders are automatically added to the list of practitioners associated with the healthcare facility. If a practitioner does not appear on the list, then that healthcare provider may not be authorized to write medical orders for patients cared for at that healthcare facility.

11.22 What is the risk of using a default practitioner in the Ordered By box?

It is risky because the healthcare team member might assume the medical order is written by the default practitioner. Excluding a default practitioner requires the healthcare team member to verify the identity of the practitioner who wrote the order.

11.23 What appears on the screen if the time to administer the medication has passed?

The charting software indicates that the medication is overdue.

11.24 What does the nurse do if she is unsure of the spelling of the name of the practitioner who wrote the medical order that she is entering into the electronic charting software?

She selects the Soundex box and then enters the phonetic spelling of the practitioner's name.

11.25 What might it mean if portions of the Order Detail screen are grayed, prohibiting the healthcare provider from entering or changing the value on the screen?

- The value cannot be changed until a previous value is entered. Once the previous value is entered, charting software ungrays the value, enabling the healthcare provider to change it.

- The value on the screen is set by default by the software. You cannot enter the value, for example, if frequency is set to Once, the duration must be 1.

- The detail does not pertain to the order.

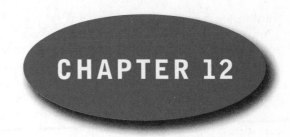

CHAPTER 12

Private Practice and Clinics

12.1   Private Practice

Private practice is a term that is used to describe an environment where care is provided by a practitioner or group of practitioners usually outside the hospital, as opposed to inpatient hospital care. This includes a single practitioner practice and a group practice where several practitioners join together and share a facility and support staff.

Private practices typically focus on providing primary health care or specialized healthcare. Some group practices might include both primary practitioners and specialists although each act independently and are joined together principally for economic reasons.

The goal of a primary-care health provider is threefold:

- Regularly monitor a patient's health and provide preventive care through annual physicals and immunizations

- Treat routine disorders

- Be a gatekeeper for medical care

A gatekeeper is a healthcare provider who assesses the patient to determine if the patient requires specialized care. If greater care is required, then the gatekeeper refers the patient to one or more specialists and coordinates care among the specialists. Third-party payers require subscribers to select a primary-care health provider to be the gatekeeper. Self-paying patients also utilize a primary-care health providers as gatekeepers.

The goal of a specialist is to provide in-depth knowledge and treatment for a narrow range of disorders that usually affect a system of the body. Patients are referred by a primary-care health provider to a specialist who sees patients to treat acute stages of particular disorders. A specialist stops seeing the patient once the acute stage is resolved, although a specialist continues to see patients who have chronic illness related to the specialty.

12.2   Private Practice and Expenses

A private practice is a small business usually owned by practitioners with the objective of making a profit. Practitioners initially invest money to lease or purchase the facility, acquire equipment, hire staff, and then attract customers to provide a revenue stream to the practice. There are two categories of customers. These are patients and third-party payers. Healthcare services are rendered to patients who directly pay a small co-payment to the private practice. Third-party payers pay the practice most of their revenue for rendering services to patients based on negotiated rates with third-party payers.

There are numerous third-party payers. Each has rules governing the type of services for which they will reimburse the practice and the amount of money paid for those services. In addition, the practice must document for third-party payers the need for the service and that the service was rendered. The practice incurs cost to adhere to these rules, which affects the profitability of the practices.

Practitioners who own a private practice are sensitive to the expenses to run the practice because each dollar spent on operating the business is less profit for the healthcare provider. A healthcare provider may feel that spending money on the business is coming directly from the healthcare provider's pocket.

12.3 Private Practice and Record Keeping

Each patient of a medical practice has a medical record. Until recently medical records consisted of file folders. Typically the healthcare provider charts by exception. The chart contains identifying information, vital signs taken at each visit, tests results, and anything unusual. The chart will also contain any prescribed treatment.

Some practitioners organize their medical records as a single-page checklist of common complaints, common tests, and common treatments. This is especially true for specialists who have built their practice around a narrow set of disorders. The healthcare provider is able to assess the patient, check the appropriate boxes, and turn the checklist over to the nurse and the practice's billing department for follow-up care and billing.

Typically a medical record in a private practice is not as voluminous as the medical record of a hospital patient, unless the patient has a chronic condition. Practitioners in private practice want to minimize the size of medical records because of the processing and storage costs. These costs directly impact the healthcare provider's profit from the practice.

A large number of patients are seen infrequently by the healthcare provider because many patients only visit the healthcare provider when home remedies don't resolve a medical complaint. Generally, patients don't go to the doctor if they feel well. Therefore, practitioners balance the cost of collecting, processing, and storing a patient's medical information with the medical, legal, and billing need for caring for the patient and holding that information for regulatory and legal requirements.

12.4 Private Practice and Electronic Medical Record Keeping

Private practices have been slow to adopt electronic medical-records software based on cost-benefit analysis. Practitioners are willing to expend money to solve a problem. For example, a medical billing and coding specialist is hired to expedite pending revenue from third-party payers. However, electronic medical records do not solve a problem for the healthcare provider, since a process is in place and working well to record patient information using paper medical records.

The cost of converting to electronic medical record keeping is relatively high. New computers must be acquired. A computer network needs to be designed and installed. Computers and the computer network require ongoing maintenance. The staff must be trained to use the computer and network. And, the practice must acquire electronic medical records software.

Acquiring EMR software is challenging because there is no single software that is standard throughout the industry. For example, Microsoft Office is the default standard for word processing, spreadsheets, and presentation software. There is no comparative product for EMR software. Further complicating the acquisition process is the fact that EMR software are not compatible with one another. That is, changing from one EMR software to another isn't easy because the format of patient information is different in each EMR software product.

Converting to EMR software and related computers is a distraction to the practice and typically requires the healthcare provider to reduce the number of daily appointments to accommodate conversion and staff training. A reduction in appointments leads to decreased revenue for the practice.

Some practices discovered that EMR software is not as efficient as paper medical records for the healthcare provider. When a healthcare provider enters the examination room, she opens a very thick file folder, reviews the patient's history, and then assesses the patient. She then writes a few words, checks a few boxes, and gives the patient a prescription. The healthcare provider then moves on to the next patient. With EMR software, the healthcare provider calls the patient's medical records to the screen and then navigates through the interface to review the patient's history. After the assessment, the healthcare provider navigates through the interface again to document the patient's visit. Navigation is more time-consuming than writing a few notes on paper. Furthermore, the healthcare provider needs to type any narrative, which is also time-consuming if the healthcare provider is not a proficient typist.

Private practices take into consideration the initial and ongoing expense of EMR software, the incompatibility of EMR software, along with the perceived inefficiencies compared with the cost. Some practices conclude that EMR software causes more problems than it solves.

12.5 Electronic Medical Record Keeping Incentive

An electronic medical record is more efficient than paper medical records once patient information is entered into the EMR software. In theory, patient's information can be electronically transferred to other practitioners, healthcare facilities, and third-party payers. In addition, EMR software and related software can analyze patient information to decrease the risk of errors and to recommend the most cost-effective treatment path for the patient. Billing and reimbursements can be seamless because data can be electronically transmitted and processed with little human intervention.

The United States Congress passed the American Recovery and Reinvestment Act of 2009 that mandated that all practitioners and healthcare facilities convert from paper medical records to electronic medical records by 2014. The government has provided financial incentives to ease the financial burden realized in the conversion process.

The goal of this provision of the American Recovery and Reinvestment Act of 2009 is to reduce Medicare and Medicaid costs for the government. Medicare and Medicaid are the largest third-party payers. EMR enables the government to automate the processing of claims and assists investigators to identify fraud.

The American Recovery and Reinvestment Act of 2009 also established a disincentive for not converting to EMR. Practitioners and healthcare facilities will lose one percent of their Medicare and Medicaid reimbursements if they fail to use an EMR by the required date. Reimbursement decreases grow incrementally to five percent in subsequent years. Healthcare practices and healthcare facilities could see their profits decrease if they do not implement EMR.

Medicare and Medicaid historically set the standard for reimbursements and processing claims. Healthcare practices that have little or no Medicare and Medicaid patients can expect other third-party payers to follow suit and therefore are likely to convert from paper to EMR in order to maintain the current level of reimbursements from third-party payers.

12.6 Ownership of Electronic Medical Record

In an ideal world, any healthcare provider can access a patient's healthcare record online regardless of who created the record and regardless of where the record is stored as long as the patient grants permission to the healthcare provider. The healthcare provider can legally access patient information without the patient's permission under certain circumstances.

In the real world, practitioners and healthcare facilities see the patient's electronic healthcare record as proprietary information that gives them the edge over the competition. Some practices and healthcare facilities believe that a patient will return to the healthcare provider who can answer their healthcare questions and address their complaints swiftly. To do this, the provider must be able to quickly access the patient's electronic medical record.

The issues of who owns a patient's medical record was resolved years ago with the passage of the Health Insurance Portability and Accountability Act (HIPAA) of 1996. The information in the medical record is owned by the patient, and therefore the patient must be given full access to the medical record and be provided a copy at no cost or a reasonable cost.

However, the healthcare provider and healthcare facility own the format of the patient's medical record. The format is the way patient information is stored in the EMR software's database and is also the physical form of the information such as an x-ray. This means the patient must be given information contained in the EMR but not necessarily the electronic format of the EMR. Simply, the patient is given a printed copy of the record and not an electronic copy because the healthcare provider or the healthcare facility owns the electronic format of the patient's medical record.

12.7 Exchanging Electronic Medical Records

The Office of the National Coordinator for Health Information Technology provides grants to government and independent organizations that provide health information exchanges. A healthcare information exchange is an electronic facility that enables sharing healthcare information with authorized providers, healthcare facilities, and ancillary organizations such as pharmacies.

The health information exchange adopts standards for requesting, transferring, and receiving electronic medical records. EMR software manufacturers are expected to incorporate features into their software to facilitate these events. The EMR software converts its data to the standard format before transmitting the data over the health information exchange. Likewise, the receiving EMR software converts the data from the standard to its own data format.

However, the exchange of health information is dependent upon the participation of EMR software manufacturers. Some widely used EMR software products are quick to incorporate transfers. Those who are not widely used might be less encouraged to build this feature into their product because of cost and the competitive climate.

12.8 Private Practice Scheduling

EMR software for private practice has a different focus than that of hospitals and other in-patient facilities because of the different requirements of a private practice. Central to operations of a private practice is scheduling of both the healthcare provider and patients. Scheduling appointments is challenging for private practice because each time slot in the schedule is expected to produce revenue for the practice. A missed appointment by either the patient or healthcare provider directly impacts the business side of the practice.

Many private-practice EMR software products have an integrated scheduling feature that enables the office staff and the healthcare provider to manage the schedules for the practice. Typically there are two schedules. One is the healthcare provider's full schedule that includes personal activities not related to the practice, and the other is the healthcare provider's practice schedule, which is time available to see patients.

The scheduling process begins with the healthcare provider entering days and times when he or she is able to see patients into the scheduling software. The staff then makes appointments with patients for those times. The healthcare provider is always able to remove unfilled appointment slots in the schedule, making them unavailable to patients without having to inform the staff because the scheduling software prevents the staff from booking appointments during those periods of time.

Likewise, the healthcare provider can enter a personal schedule into the scheduling software enabling her to see her complete schedule. Personal schedules can be shared with or hidden from the staff depending on the preference of the healthcare provider. A hidden personal schedule appears as unavailable time if viewed by the staff, and details are available only to the healthcare provider.

Scheduling software defaults to 15-minute appointments, however the length of the appointment can be changed to suit the needs of the practice. If a patient needs more time, then the staff books two adjacent time slots to extend the appointment.

The staff can also use the scheduling software to record the time that the patient checked into the office, the examining room assigned to the patient, the reason for the visit, and the checkout time. This tells the healthcare provider if the patient is in the waiting room or has moved into the examination room and in which examination room she'll find the patient.

More sophisticated scheduling software can forecast patient traffic based on information entered into the schedule. For example, it can project the wait time for patients if the healthcare provider is late for an appointment or spends more than the scheduled time with a patient. Scheduling software can also project the number of patients who keep appointments and which patients don't keep appointments, enabling the staff to book accordingly.

Scheduling software links to patient information, which is beneficial because the healthcare provider can select the patient from the schedule and the EMR software automatically displays the patient's medical record on the screen. In addition, some scheduling software can link to programs that automatically send reminders to patients via e-mails or with computer-generated phone calls.

12.9 The Dashboard

Practitioners in private practice use a screen referred to as a dashboard to help manage their time and work. The name *dashboard* comes from the dashboard of a car. The dashboard provides a synopsis of all information needed to operate the car, such as the speed, amount of fuel, and whether or not a door is open.

The EMR dashboard has a similar purpose for the practice. At the top of the dashboard (Figure 12.1) is the schedule listing patient appointments and related information. There is a message board where the staff can communicate with the healthcare provider without having to interrupt him or her. There is a to-do list used by the staff and the healthcare provider to remind the healthcare provider of pending activities.

The Lab Review section of the dashboard lists available lab results that the healthcare provider needs to review. She can select the item and the software displays the lab results on the screen if the results are transmitted electronically. Otherwise, the healthcare provider needs to physically review the paper results.

Some practitioners dictate progress and summary notes about a patient that are then typed by a medical transcriber. The transcription is then electronically transmitted to the healthcare provider for review and notices of the transcription appear in the Note Review section of the dashboard. The healthcare provider selects the item, and the note is displayed on the screen.

Some dashboards include a financial feature that enables the healthcare provider to review the practice's financial status. The financial status includes co-pays, reimbursements received, pending reimbursements, and possibly expenses. This is particularly useful in a single-provider private practice or a practice where the healthcare provider is one of the owners.

12.10 The Patient's Chart

The patient's electronic chart is designed for the needs of the private practice in that information is organized into convenient tabs with the focus of providing the patient with outpatient services. Figure 12.2 is an example of a chart used in a private practice. Notice that the Chart Summary is the first tab and is usually the initial entry point for the healthcare provider because this tab gives an overview of the patient. The Progress Notes tab follows, enabling the healthcare provider to read the sequence of events that recently occurred with the patient.

Tabs related to the patient's history are grouped into a section of the chart. These include medical, social, and family history giving the clinician clues to better understand the patient's needs and treatments to address the patient's complaint. The left column of the chart continues with tabs that focus on consults, discharge summary, letters, orders, and other elements. A colored marker appears in the corner of the tab indicating that the tab contains information. Most tabs don't contain information because many patients have acute rather than chronic problems that are resolved in a couple of visits.

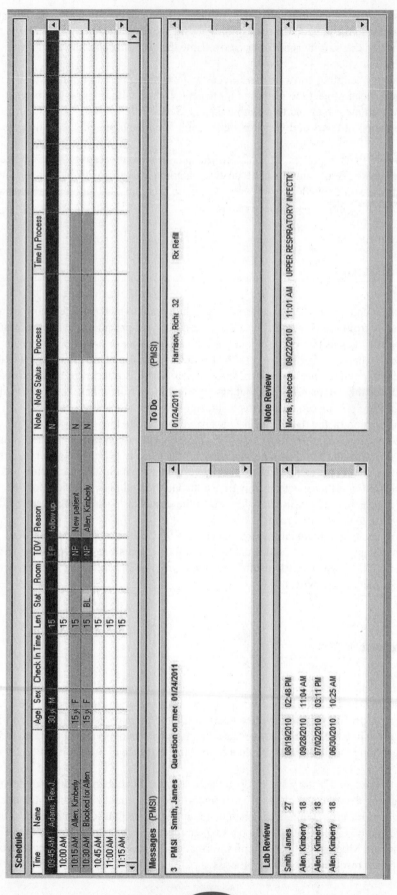

Figure 12.1

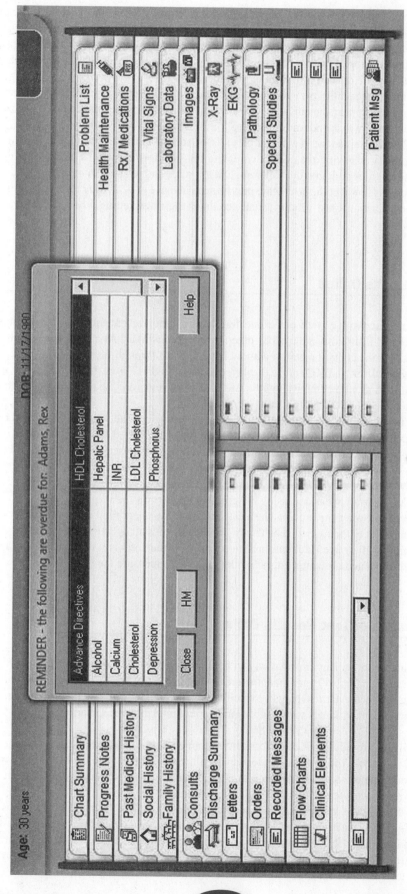

Figure 12.2

The first section on the right side of the chart contains information that is most useful to the practitioners. These are the patient's problem list, health maintenance record, and prescription and medications.

The second section lists measurements and test results including vital signs, lab data, x-rays and other images, EKGs, and results from biopsies and other tissue studies. There is also a section for Special Studies that is a catch tab for tests that are outside the realm of the other tabs.

Notice that the more frequently used tabs are at the top of each column and the less-used tabs are toward the bottom. A color marker appears on tabs that have content. This enables the healthcare provide to easily navigate the chart without having to spend time searching for information.

Some EMR software reminds the healthcare provider of actions that are overdue for the patient. This can include ordering lab tests or having the patient complete missing forms, such as an advance directive. The reminder is generated by rules built into the software. Default rules and related recommended actions are set by the software manufacturer; however the healthcare provider can activate or deactivate rules depending on the preference of the practice. The software vendor usually changes the rules setting when the software is initially installed.

12.11 Test Results Online

EMR software can interface with clinical electronic devices and import test results from other resources such as healthcare exchanges and EMR software used by other healthcare facilities. As a result, the healthcare provider can display test results at the click of a button without having to sift through files of paper.

For example, the results of an EKG can be displayed as illustrated in Figure 12.3. The display shows administrative information such as who administered the EKG and who reviewed the results along with the patient's blood pressure at the time the EKG was given.

In addition, the EKG strip is shown enabling the healthcare provider to analyze the results and reach her own diagnosis. In the upper middle section of the screen is the computer-generated diagnosis of the EKG strip. In this example, the EKG is normal. Typically, the healthcare provider will make her own diagnosis and then compare this to the diagnosis of the computer. The healthcare provider will delete the computer's diagnosis, add her own diagnosis, or modify the computer's diagnosis according to the healthcare provider's preference.

Waves on an EKG strip are measured using the grid that appears on the strip. The software measures EKG waves for the healthcare provider and presents the measurement in the upper right corner of the screen to the right of the diagnosis. This reduces the time the healthcare provider spends analyzing the wave. Once the healthcare provider is confident that the waves are measured accurately by the software, then the focus can be directed toward the computer-generated measurement rather than having to measure the EKG waves herself.

12.12 Challenges of Test Results Online

Not all test results and other patient information can be imported into EMR private-practice software because of incompatible features among software manufactures. Although there are efforts for practitioners and facilities to use electronic healthcare data exchanges to facilitate the interchange of patient information, some healthcare facilities and private practitioners view exchanging patient information as sharing proprietary information with a competitor.

As an alternative to providing patient information in an electronic form that can be retained by another healthcare provider in his own EMR, some vendors and healthcare facilities give the healthcare provider access to their own EMR and related software applications. This means that the healthcare provider can remotely log into the other software to view test results and patient information.

This alternative facilitates exchange of patient information but does not necessarily allow the patient's information to be imported into another EMR system. This forces the private-practice healthcare provider to learn how to use different EMR and related software. That is, each vendor and each healthcare facility can have different software. This can be troublesome, especially in metropolitan areas where there are several hospitals that provide tests and in-patient services to patients of private practice practitioners.

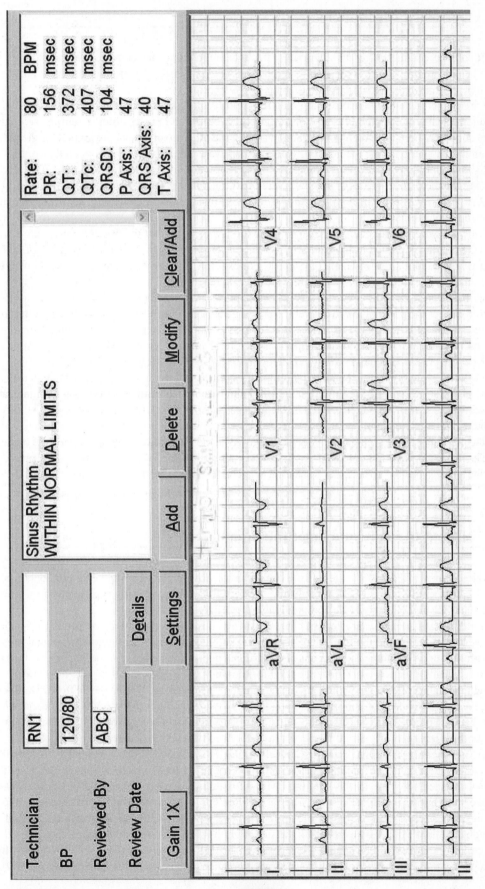

Figure 12.3

189

12.13 Electronic Prescriptions

Many EMR software products offer private-practice healthcare providers an electronic prescription feature that enables the healthcare provider to write the prescription into the prescription section of the EMR software and then automatically transmits the prescription to the patient's pharmacy.

There are numerous advantages to using electronic prescriptions. The most important is that the EMR software automatically checks the prescription for conflicts before the prescription is sent to the pharmacy. Conflicts occur when there is a potential interaction among the other medications prescribed for the patient or if the patient has an allergy to the medication. The EMR software displays a warning when the conflict is discovered as shown in Figure 12.4. In this example, a prescriber wrote a prescription for amoxicillin. The EMR software searched the patient's records and discovered that the patient is allergic to amoxicillin. The warning message alerts the prescriber to the conflict and lists reactions that patient might experience if the patient takes the prescribed medication.

The EMR software permits the prescriber to write the prescription, but the prescriber is likely to receive a call from the pharmacy related to the conflict. The prescriber must weigh the patient's benefit of taking the medication vs. the patient's risk of an allergic attack. For example, the prescriber may decide to prescribe the medication and another medication to counteract the allergic reaction.

Another benefit of electronic prescriptions is that the prescription is electronically transferred to the pharmacy. No longer does the patient have to deliver the prescription. There is much efficiency realized through this process. The uppermost is security. This reduces the likelihood that the patient will lose the prescription or that a prescription might be a fraud. Errors are reduced as the prescription is legible, and the pharmacist no longer has to interpret the prescriber's handwriting or call the prescriber for clarification.

EMR software typically have a template or templates built-in that the healthcare provider can use, reducing the time necessary to write a prescription. Typically a prescriber has a set of medications that are ordered for diagnoses that he sees in the practice. Each medication has a name, dose, frequency, and route. All this information is built-in to the template.

Once the prescriber creates the set, then only medications in the set appear in the look-up feature of the EMR software. The prescriber then selects the appropriate medication and the EMR software fills in the prescription. The prescriber always has the opportunity to change whatever is written on the prescription.

12.14 Tailoring the Software and Staff Training

The lack of uniformity of EMR software poses a challenge for private practice healthcare providers who need to have staff competent to interact with the software. EMR software is similar to yet different from word processing, spreadsheet, and other software commonly used in offices.

The similarities are graphic-user interface elements such as push buttons, drop-down menus, pop-up menus, check boxes, radio buttons, and the like. Many employees know how to interact with software that uses these elements with little or no training. This was one of the original goals of the graphic-user interface designs in that over time the standard interface will reduce the need for training.

Although the staff probably knows how to use the interface elements, navigating the EMR software remains a challenge because of the lack of uniformity among EMR software products. Most EMR software products do provide for the same functionality and probably use standard medical terminology to record patient information. However, the organization of patient information differs, as seen throughout chapters of this book.

Further complicating training is the fact that many EMR software products are tailored to the client. Tailoring is a technique software manufacturers use to meet specific needs of a client without the client having to develop customized software. In this way the EMR software is like a business suit. The client can ask the tailor to make him a business suit. The result is a perfectly fitted suit at an expensive price. Alternatively, the client can buy a business suit off the rack that is the correct general size, and then the tailor adjusts the suit to fit. Depending on the client's build, adjustments to the suit might be sufficient and at a reasonable price.

Many private practices and healthcare facilities license EMR software products with the hopes that the product is a perfect fit. EMR software manufacturers are continuously redesigning and upgrading their products,

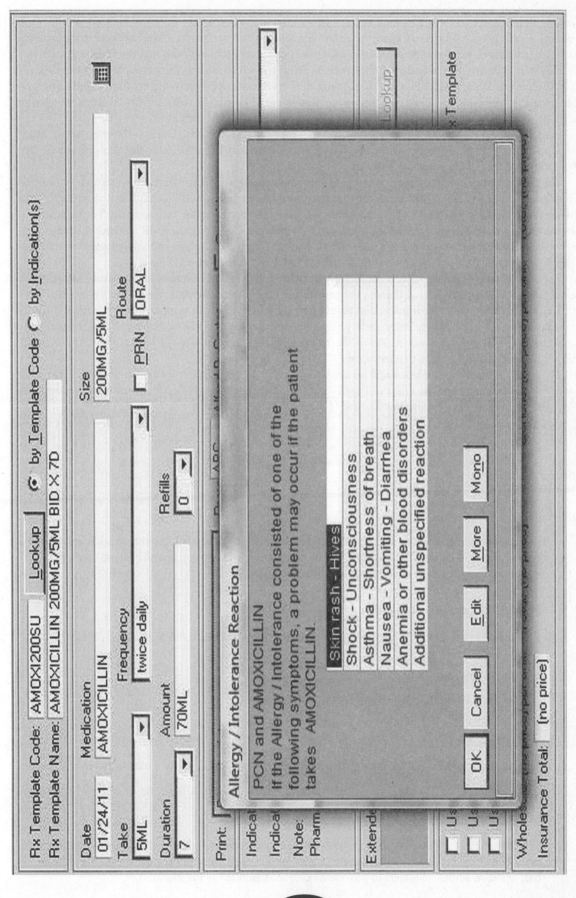

Figure 12.4

191

incorporating features requested by their customers with the goal to avoid or minimize the need to tailor their products. Every private practice is faced with the same operational problems. EMR software manufacturers would like to believe they have the solution to all those operational problems built into the EMR software.

However, clients often have already implemented their own solutions to those operational problems and are typically confronted with a dilemma. Do they change the way the practice operates to conform to the EMR software product's methodology? If so, then there is no need to modify the EMR software. Or, do they seek to tailor the EMR software to conform to their operation? If so, then the initial cost increases.

Each private practice and healthcare facility decides the best approach based on good business sense. Many decide to tailor the EMR software to their operational needs. Two major drawbacks to this decision are the cost of tailoring and the required ongoing training.

The tailoring process requires one or more analysts who know the EMR software product to assess the operational needs of the practice. These needs are then translated into instructions for technicians to then modify the EMR software accordingly. Think of the analyst as the tailor who marks up the business suit. The technician is the seamstress who makes changes to the business suit. Sometimes modifying the EMR software is costly, especially when the off-the-rack suit doesn't fit the client's build. That is, the client's operational needs are dramatically different from the operational rules built into the EMR software product.

The costs of tailoring can escalate unpredictably because each time the client sees the modified EMR software the client tends to ask for additional changes to the software. Each change increases the cost of the product.

Tailored EMR software also impacts staff training. Initially, the entire staff is trained when the EMR software product is adopted by the practice. Subsequently, the office manager looks to hire candidates who are familiar with that particular EMR software product. This is like hiring staff who know how to use Microsoft Word and Excel. There is no need to train them on that software.

The reality is that the candidate might be already trained to use the EMR software but not with a particular practice's modifications. The candidate still needs to learn to navigate the modified EMR software product. This delays the time before the new employee is fully functional in the position.

Solved Problems

12.1   What is a private practice?

Private practice is a term that is used to describe a healthcare facility that provides healthcare outside a hospital setting. This includes a single practitioner practice and a group practice where several practitioners join together and share a facility and support staff.

12.2   What are the goals of a private practice?

- To regularly monitor a patient's health and provide preventive care through annual physicals and immunizations

- To treat routine disorders

- To be gatekeepers for medical care

12.3   What is the goal of a specialist private practice?

The goal of a specialist is to provide in-depth knowledge and treatment for a narrow range of disorders that usually affect a system of the body.

12.4   How is a private practice a business?

A private practice is a small business usually owned by practitioners with the objective of making a profit. Practitioners initially invest money to lease or purchase the facility, acquire equipment, hire staff, and then attract customers to provide a revenue stream to the practice.

12.5 Who are the customers of a private practice?

There are two categories of customers: these are patients and third-party payers.

12.6 Why do private practices want to minimize the size of medical records?

Practitioners in private practice want to minimize the size of medical records because of processing and storage costs.

12.7 What steps are needed convert a private practice to EMR software products?

New computers must be acquired. A computer network needs to be designed and installed. Computers and the computer network must be maintained on a regular basis. The staff must be trained to use the computer and network, and the practice must acquire electronic medical record software.

12.8 What is the standard EMR software product for private practice?

There is no standard EMR software product.

12.9 Why is EMR software sometimes less efficient than paper charts in a private practice?

EMR software is sometimes considered less efficient for private-practice practitioners when the clinician must document a patient. Paper medical records enable the clinician to open a file folder, write a progress note, and check results of the patient assessment. EMR software requires the clinician to navigate through computer screens to document the patient's visit, which can be time-consuming.

12.10 Why is EMR software more efficient than paper charts in a private practice?

Patient information entered into EMR software requires less storage space than paper charts and can be retrieved quickly even from remote locations. Furthermore, patient information can be electronically transmitted to other healthcare facilities and to third-party payers decreasing the reimbursement time.

12.11 Why would a private practice avoid adopting EMR software?

A private practice is a small business where a primary objective is for the healthcare provider to minimize expenses in an effort to increase profits. EMR software products and related technology are expensive to acquire and maintain when compared to the cost of paper charts. Therefore, the additional expense of EMR software products may not be perceived as a wise business decision.

12.12 Why would a private practice adopt EMR software?

The American Recovery and Reinvestment Act of 2009 mandates that all practitioners use electronic medical records by 2014, and the government has provided financial grants to lessen the financial burden of the initial implementation of the EMR products and related equipment.

12.13 What occurs if a private practice does not adopt EMR software?

The private practice will lose one percent of their Medicare and Medicaid reimbursement if they fail to use EMR software. Reimbursements decrease incrementally growing to five percent in subsequent years.

12.14 Why is there a penalty for not adopting EMR software?

The goal is to reduce Medicare and Medicaid cost for the government by automating claims processing and assisting investigations of identify fraud.

12.15   Why would a private practice adopt EMR software if they don't service Medicare and Medicaid patients?

Medicare and Medicaid historically set the standard for reimbursements and processing claims. Healthcare practices that have little or no Medicare and Medicaid patients can expect other third-party payers to follow suit and therefore are likely to need to convert from paper to EMR in order to maintain the current level of reimbursements from third-party payers.

12.16   Who owns a patient's electronic medical record?

The private practice and healthcare facility owns the format of the patient's medical record, and the patient has the right to see and acquire a copy of the content of the patient's medical record.

12.17   What is a format of an electronic medical record?

The format of an electronic medical record is the way the medical record is organized on electronic media.

12.18   How does the format differ from the content of an electronic medical record?

The content is the actual information about the patient stored in the electronic medical record. The format is the way that information is organized and stored on the computer.

12.19   How are medical records exchanged among practitioners?

The Office of the National Coordinator for Health Information Technology provides grants to government and independent organizations that provide health information exchanges. A healthcare information exchange is an electronic facility that enables sharing healthcare information with authorized providers, healthcare facilities, and ancillary organizations such as pharmacies.

12.20   What factor impedes sharing a patient's electronic medical records among practitioners?

Practitioners view a patient's electronic medical record as proprietary information that gives the healthcare provider a business advantage over competing practitioners. Therefore, some practitioners are hesitant to share patient information electronically with other practitioners.

12.21   What is a key element in private-practice EMR software products that are not usually found in hospital EMR software products?

Appointment scheduling is a key feature in private practice EMR software products that is not typically found in hospital EMR software products.

12.22   Where does the patient scheduling process begin in a private practice?

Scheduling begins when the healthcare provider blocks time in the scheduling software to see patients.

12.23   What is a dashboard?

A dashboard is a feature of EMR software products for private practice that provides a synopsis of information for the healthcare provider. It lists the day's schedule and related information about appointments and also includes a message board, to-do list, and lab results that need to be reviewed.

12.24   What is a drawback to viewing test results online?

In a private practice, tests might be performed by other practitioners and at other facilities. Results may not be electronically transferable to the private practice's EMR software. Results may be available online; however the healthcare provider might need to access test results using the other party's EMR software.

12.25   What is the advantage of using electronic prescriptions?

- EMR software automatically checks the prescription for conflicts with a patient's other current medications and with the patient's allergies.

- Prescriptions electronically transferred to the pharmacy increase security and reduce the likelihood that the patient will lose the prescription.

- The prescription is legible, and the pharmacist no longer has to interpret the prescriber's handwriting or call the prescriber for clarification.

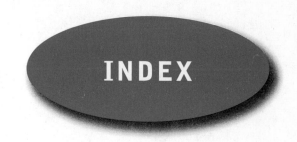

INDEX

Note: The letters *f* or *t* following page numbers refer to figures or tables, respectively.